The Genetics and Epidemiology of Inflammatory Bowel Disease

Frontiers of Gastrointestinal Research

Vol. 11

Series Editor
P. Rozen, Tel Aviv

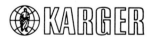 KARGER

Basel · München · Paris · London · New York · New Delhi · Singapore · Tokyo · Sydney

The Genetics and Epidemiology of Inflammatory Bowel Disease

Volume Editors
R. McConnell, Liverpool
P. Rozen, Tel Aviv
M. Langman, Nottingham
T. Gilat, Tel Aviv

62 figures and 68 tables, 1986

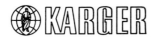

Basel · München · Paris · London · New York · New Delhi · Singapore · Tokyo · Sydney

Frontiers of Gastrointestinal Research

National Library of Medicine, Cataloging in Publication
 The Genetics and epidemiology of inflammatory
 bowel disease / volume editors, R. McConnell [et al.]. – Basel;
 New York: Karger, 1986.
 (Frontiers of gastrointestinal research; vol. 11)
 Based on an international meeting held in Liverpool in 1984.
 Includes index.
 1. Colitis, Ulcerative – familial & genetic – congresses
 2. Colitis, Ulcerative – occurrence – congresses
 3. Crohn Disease – familial & genetic congresses
 4. Crohn Disease – occurrence – congresses
 I. McConnell, Richard B. II. Series
 W1 FR946E v. 11 [WI 522 G328 1984]

 ISBN 3-8055-4265-8

Drug Dosage

The authors and the publisher have exerted every effort to ensure that drug selection and dosage set forth in this text are in accord with current recommendations and practice at the time of publication. However, in view of ongoing research, changes in government regulations, and the constant flow of information relating to drug therapy and drug reactions, the reader is urged to check the package insert for each drug for any change in indications and dosage and for added warnings and precautions. This is particularly important when the recommended agent is a new and/or infrequently employed drug.

© Copyright 1986 by S. Karger AG, P.O. Box. CH-4009 Basel (Switzerland)
 Printed in Switzerland by Thür AG Offsetdruck, Pratteln
 ISBN 3-8055-4265-8

Contents

Time Trends

Ethnic, Religious and Occupational Groups

Predisposing Factors

Preface

It is a clinical cliche to describe the occurrence of chronic inflammatory bowel disease as being the result of the interplay of genetic and environmental factors. But, however obvious the interplay may be, we need
to define the responsible factors. By defining the genetic influences we
may gain insight into the mechanisms and by defining the more and the
less susceptible we may make it easier to establish which environmental
factors are responsible for causing the disease. Epidemiological studies
can be broadly of two types, they can describe the characteristics of
populations, and so define groups at-risk, consequently generating
hypotheses on causation, or they may be directed at establishing whether
suggestions made about causation are indeed well founded.

This volume brings together a series of reviews of genetic and environmental factors influencing the liability to ulcerative colitis and
Crohn's disease. They cover the full field of study, and range from
accounts of the frequency of disease in families, in special groups such as
children or migrants, and in geographic areas of special interest where
studies have been infrequent, such as Southern Europe, to considerations
of specific factors associated with disease such as smoking habits. In the
prevailing state of uncertainty about causes, the data are predominantly
descriptive in nature; however, we believe that they can also be described
fairly as being comprehensive. They arise as the product of an international meeting held in Liverpool in 1984 and we think that the information provides a sound basis upon which anyone seeking to extend our
knowledge of Crohn's disease and ulcerative colitis could build.

The editors

Genetic Studies

Front. gastrointest. Res., vol. 11, pp. 1–11 (Karger, Basel 1986)

Inflammatory Bowel Disease:
A Review of Previous Genetic Studies and the
Liverpool Family Data

R. B. McConnell, Joan M. Shaw, Elizabeth J. Whibley,
T. H. McConnell

Department of Medicine, University of Liverpool and Royal Liverpool and
Broadgreen Hospitals, Liverpool, UK

It is interesting that the very first observations of ileitis made by
Crohn [1], 50 years ago, were on a 14-year-old boy whose 32-year-old
sister developed the condition soon afterwards. *Crohn* commented that
'the occurrence may be purely accidental or it may have significance as
to a congenital predisposition or a transmissable causative agent in this
disease'.

Familial ulcerative colitis had been reported early in this century [2]
and there have been numerous reports since then of inflammatory bowel
disease occurring in an isolated family. Only rarely are such reports of
value in interpreting the genetic aspects of the condition. With a disease
which is moderately common in the population, quite large family aggre-
gations can be expected by chance alone. However, some clues to the
genetic basis of the condition can be gained by the types of intra-familial
relationship and their relative frequencies. Perhaps the main value of
these reports has been the frequency of the reports of the occurrence,
in the same family, of both Crohn's disease and ulcerative colitis.

Distribution of Cases within Families

Kirsner [3] described the many reports, in the literature, of three or
more members of the same family with inflammatory bowel disease.
Table I is a compilation of the reports of familial cases of inflammatory
bowel disease up to 1977. It will be noted that parent-child and sib-sib
combinations have been reported much more commonly than more dis-
tant relatives. It will also be noted that, as well as familial occurrences of
ulcerative colitis and Crohn's disease, there is a column enumerating the
reports of both diseases in the same family. These reports are of little

Table I. Familial occurrences reported before 1978

	Ulcerative colitis	Crohn's disease	Mixed ulcerative colitis and Crohn's disease
Parent-offspring	43	18	7
Sib-sib	51	27	12
Collateral relatives	13	14	9
Twins			
Concordant	5	7	0
Discordant	6	1	0
Husband and wife	1	1	1

statistical value as it seems likely that a clinician would report such an occurrence when he would not report a family with 2 cases of ulcerative colitis or 2 cases of Crohn's disease. In the earlier reports there may have been room for doubts of the diagnoses, but this explanation gradually became untenable especially when a very large family aggregation, with several cases of both ulcerative colitis and Crohn's disease, was reported [4].

Of greater value than the compilation of various reports in table I is the detailed single-series, New York data, presented by *Korelitz* [5]. Because they are all from his own patients they give the distribution of intrafamilial relationships free from the possible bias of the irregular ascertainment of isolated reports. His 353 index patients all had Crohn's disease and 72 of them (20.4%) had one or more relatives who also suffered with Crohn's disease or ulcerative colitis. The parent-offspring occurrences were slightly more frequent than sib-sib combinations, and the number of affected first cousins, uncles and aunts are much greater than the previous reports in the literature had indicated. Even though *Korelitz* found as many as 8 affected people in one family, there is nothing in his data to suggest either dominant or recessive inheritance, nor even of a major gene contribution. They are in keeping with quantitative, multifactorial heredity rather than the familial occurrences being due entirely to the common family environment.

The Cleveland Clinic data [6] are not quite comparable with those of *Korelitz* [5] as the single series of 838 inflammatory bowel disease patients had all had an onset of the disease before 21 years of age. It can be seen that the number of affected parents was more than the number of affected sibs but because of the youth of the propositi, more sibs may subsequently develop the disease. On the whole, however, these Cleveland data lend support to *Korelitz's* data and to an interpretation of polygenic inheritance.

Table II. Inflammatory bowel disease among first-degree relatives of 336 Liverpool patients with Crohn's disease or ulcerative colitis

	Ulcerative colitis patients (n = 171)	Crohn's disease patients (n = 165)
With affected relative	20	31
1 generation only affected	13	17
2 generations affected	7	14
Relationships		
Father-offspring	2	6
Mother-offspring	5	8
Sib-sib	16	27
Number of relatives		
Parents	342	330
Sibs	533	487
Offspring	251	254

Study of the families of 336 Liverpool IBD families has given rather different results, as can be seen in table II. It can be seen that sib-sib combinations have been found very much more frequently than parent-sib combinations, compared with the preponderance of parent-sib combinations in the New York and Cleveland data. This difference may be partly accounted for by the number of families in the Liverpool series which contained several affected sibs and therefore contributed multiple sib-sib relationships. One male Crohn's patient had his father and a brother affected by Crohn's disease and a brother and a sister with ulcerative colitis, whilst a female Crohn's patient had 4 affected sisters. Though the Liverpool study has shown a marked same-generation distribution there is again no evidence of strong single-gene inheritance and these data are in fact, more suggestive of polygenic or infective influence.

Twins

The reports of twins up to 1978 is listed in table I. It can be seen that amongst the monozygotic twins there is a high concordance rate for Crohn's disease (7 of 8) but not for ulcerative colitis (5 of 11). It is difficult to imagine a reason why clinicians should report a pair of twins when only one has ulcerative colitis more readily, than a pair when only one is affected by Crohn's disease. Therefore, these data support the theory that heredity is more important in Crohn's disease than in ulcerative colitis.

There has been another report of discordance in identical twins in which one had ulcerative colitis [7]. Also, a report of a pair of monozygotic twin boys who developed Crohn's disease affecting the terminal ileum, colon and rectum, within 8 months of each other, when 14 years of age [8]. The authors considered 11 reported sets of twins with Crohn's disease and state that all became symptomatic within 6 years of each other and in seven instances the interval of onset between the twins was less than 1 year. Four pairs had been raised in the same environment but in two pairs they were living apart, one pair for 10 years [9].

It is interesting that there has not yet been a report of twins, one with Crohn's disease and the other with ulcerative colitis, even though the two diseases are so often found in sib pairs and in parent-child combinations. This is further strong evidence of the two diseases having a quantitative genetic relationship.

Spouses

It will be noted in table I that up to 1978 there had been three instances of husband and wife affected, and since then five more have been reported [5, 10–13]. It is interesting that sometimes one spouse had Crohn's disease and the other ulcerative colitis. This might be interpreted as indicating that the two conditions have the same exogenous aetiology, but more probably it has been a chance occurrence. One such reported instance [13] was particularly remarkable in that first the woman developed ulcerative colitis, then 7 years later her son developed ulcerative proctitis and 2 years after that the boy's father developed Crohn's disease of the distal ileum.

Positive Family History

The numbers of people with a positive family history in reported series of inflammatory bowel disease patients has been very variable, usually between 10 and 20% being found [3]. *Paulley* [14] studied the family history of 169 London cases of ulcerative colitis and found that 19 (11.3%) had an affected first-degree relative. His controls of 98 other patients had only 2 sibs with ulcerative colitis. In a different study [15], a smaller percentage of the patients were reported as having a positive family history, but in this and other series the patients were not specially interviewed as they had been by *Paulley*. When the relatives are interviewed, the percentage found to have inflammatory bowel disease can be

Table III. Inflammatory bowel disease – affected relatives [adapted from ref. 16]

Disease	Number of patients	Numbers with positive family	Disease in relatives	
			ulcerative colitis	Crohn's disease
Ulcerative colitis	1084	66	75	13
Crohn's disease	185	20	9	12

expected to be higher than when only the patients are questioned. People can be quite ignorant of the state of health of even their own brothers and sisters in other towns.

The data from Kirsner's clinic in Chicago [16] (table III) are much more valuable and show several features which are of interest. One is that out of the 1,084 cases of ulcerative colitis there were only 66 (6.1%) with a positive family history, whilst with Crohn's disease, 20 out of 185 (10.8%) had a positive family history. It would thus appear that Crohn's disease is more often familial than ulcerative colitis. The other thing to notice in the data is that amongst the affected relatives of those with either disease there are many with the other condition. There are 13 ulcerative colitis patients with relatives affected by Crohn's disease and amongst the Crohn's disease there are 9 who had relatives with ulcerative colitis. Later, *Kirsner* [3] reported that of 103 families with more than one case of inflammatory bowel disease, 31 had both Crohn's disease and ulcerative colitis. The differential diagnosis of Crohn's disease and ulcerative colitis can be difficult and there may be uncertainty about the diagnosis in relatives. Even so, there can be no doubt that many families have had members with both definite Crohn's disease affecting the small bowel and definite colitis confined to the colon and with no features of Crohn's disease.

The data from the Cleveland Clinic [6] related only to patients with an onset of disease before the age of 21. Of the 316 ulcerative colitis patients, they found that no less than 29% had a positive family history of inflammatory bowel disease. In Crohn's disease it was even higher, 35% having a positive family history. In both diseases there was an unusually high incidence of affected second-degree relatives including grandparents. This high incidence of positive family history is very much what one finds in early onset cases of diseases in which the genetic basis involves a number of different genes, in other words a polygenic basis. For instance, patients in whom duodenal ulcer develops under the age of 15 have a very high incidence of duodenal ulcer in the parents, very often on both sides

Table IV. Results of study of families of 348 Liverpool patients: numbers of patients with a positive family history (FH) of inflammatory bowel disease (IBD) in first- or second-degree relatives, and the numbers with at least one first-degree relative affected, with the conditions found in the first-degree relatives

Proband's condition	Ulcerative colitis	Crohn's disease	IBD unclassified
Number studied	171	165	12
Positive FH of IBD			
Number	25	35	1
Percentage	14.6	21.2	8.3
Probands with first-degree relatives affected			
Number	20	31	1
Percentage	11.7	18.8	8.3
Condition of relatives:			
Ulcerative colitis	17	19	1
Crohn's disease	2	21	0
IBD	4	2	0

of the family [17]. Similarly, these young-onset inflammatory bowel disease patients at the Cleveland Clinic have a strong familial component.

Table IV shows data from Broadgreen Hospital and the Colon Clinic of the Royal Liverpool Hospital, in which the patients were investigated in some detail and the relatives interviewed. The results show the same trends as those in Chicago. Amongst the 171 ulcerative colitis patients there were 25 (14.6%) who had inflammatory bowel disease in their relatives, whilst in the 165 Crohn's patients 35 (21.2%) had affected relatives. Again, note this higher incidence of positive family history amongst the Crohn's disease patients. Again there was the mixture of ulcerative colitis and Crohn's disease in the relatives. It can be seen that among the affected relatives of the Crohn's patients there were 18 who had ulcerative colitis, but there were only 3 cases of Crohn's disease in the 30 affected relatives of the colitics. These data indicate that the reports in the literature of both conditions in one family reflect a frequent occurrence.

The data in table V show that in the Liverpool family study no significant differences were found between the patients with a positive family history and those who had no known affected relative. In particular, the patients with an affected relative, who might be expected to have a stronger genetic component in their aetiology, had not an earlier age at onset nor a more severe, nor more extensive disease than the non-familial cases.

Table V. Analysis of 336 Liverpool IBD patients

	Family history of IBD					
	Crohn's disease			ulcerative colitis		
	no	FH	%	no	FH	%
Total	165	35	21.2	171	25	14.6
Males	58	12	20.7	67	8	11.9
Females	107	23	21.5	104	17	16.3
Age at onset, years						
0–25	83	19	22.9	68	9	13.2
26–99	82	16	19.5	103	16	15.5
Extent						
Small bowel	27	6	22.2	0	0	–
Small bowel + colon	68	13	19.1	0	0	–
Colon only	57	13	22.8	171	25	14.6
Anus affected	47	10	21.3	8	1	12.5
Religion						
Protestant	93	19	20.4	91	9	9.9
Catholic	51	6	11.8	55	11	20.0
Jewish	5	5	100.0	3	1	33.3
Complications	56	8	14.3	59	11	18.6
None	111	26	23.4	121	14	11.6
Remissions	50	10	20.0	99	16	16.2
None	115	25	21.7	72	9	12.5
Severity						
Mild	40	8	20.0	76	9	11.8
Moderate	42	8	19.0	55	10	18.2
Severe	83	19	22.9	40	6	15.0

There have been a number of reports of relatives who have developed the same type or distribution of disease or perhaps the same complication. For instance, dilatation of the colon has occurred in 2 relatives with Crohn's disease [18]. This might suggest a familial tendency to this infrequent complication, but to establish whether or not this is so will entail a detailed clinical comparison of familial cases within large series of patients. This seems to have been done in a study of 10 families in which 32 cases of inflammatory bowel disease had developed [7]. It was noted that 3 of 4 affected sibpairs, who had identical HLA haplotypes, had similar disease patterns. The remaining HLA identical pair had one sib with Crohn's disease of the small bowel and the other with classical ulcerative

Table VI. Possible bases of the familial relationship of ulcerative colitis and Crohn's disease

Genetic	Environmental		Fit with data
Different	different		no
Same	different		poor
Different	same		poor
Same	same		poor
	⎰ same		poor
Shared	⎨ different		possible
	⎱ 2 factors		best

Shared = Crohn's disease developing with fuller genotype, ulcerative colitis with partial genotype; 2 factors = one for inflammatory bowel disease and another additive for Crohn's disease.

colitis. In 6 of the 10 families, the affected either all had Crohn's disease or all had ulcerative colitis. In the remaining 4 families, both diseases were found.

Thus, there is now a considerable body of evidence in favour of the relationship of the two conditions, with each other, having a genetic basis. It would appear that most likely explanation of the association of Crohn's disease and ulcerative colitis is that there is one genotype, with perhaps 10 or 15 genes, which makes people liable to develop inflammatory bowel disease. If a person has only a few of these genes, they are more liable to develop ulcerative colitis: if they have many of these genes (a more complete genotype), the clinical and pathological picture that develops is more likely to be Crohn's disease. This would explain why the relatives of people with Crohn's disease are much more likely to have inflammatory bowel disease than relatives of people with ulcerative colitis. If a patient has a large number of these genes, his or her relatives are more likely to have a moderate number of the genes than are the relatives of a patient with only a moderate number of them. In our present state of knowledge this would appear to be the most likely explanation of the familial pattern.

Environment and Heredity

The possibility cannot be ruled out that the reason for the occurrence of Crohn's disease and ulcerative colitis in the same family is not genetic, but rather that it is due to both conditions having the same environmental cause. If this were the case, a much more even geographical distribution of these two diseases would be expected. What evidence there is suggests that the incidence of ulcerative colitis is fairly uniform in the western world, whereas Crohn's disease has a more variable incidence. Also, if the two diseases had the same environmental cause, why should the incidence of Crohn's disease have increased so dramatically in the past half century, while that of ulcerative colitis remains static or may even be declining? A speculative reply might be that an environmental factor(s) that causes ulcerative colitis is gradually being replaced by a different environmental factor(s) that causes Crohn's disease. Nevertheless, the possibility cannot be ruled out that they do, in fact, have the same primary cause and that the rising incidence of Crohn's disease is due to a second additive environmental cause. This would account for the apparent trend toward replacement of ulcerative colitis by Crohn's disease in some localities. It would also possibly explain why many clinicians, including the author, have patients who 10 years ago had all the criteria of ulcerative colitis and who now have Crohn's disease.

If the two diseases have different exogenous causes, their relationship in families must have a genetic basis. This does not of course, imply that they are wholly genetically determined. It is a sound working hypothesis that all diseases that do not have a simple mendelian pattern of inheritance are due to a mixture of environmental causes acting on people of varying susceptibility, this susceptibility being genetically determined. Such states are difficult to analyse as both the environmental cause and the genetic susceptibility can vary quantitatively. In some patients heredity is the more important factor: in others a large environmental attack may be the main cause. In both ulcerative colitis and Crohn's disease, the weight of evidence points to both environment and heredity being involved in the aetiology. The various possible explanations are summarised in table VI.

Until discovery of the cause of the disease makes everything clear, the explanation most able to explain all the data is that inflammatory bowel disease is due to environmental factors which operate in some communities more than in others, and that the people who are most likely to develop it are those genetically predisposed.

Conclusions

Familial ulcerative colitis has been noted throughout this century and Crohn's disease is found in close relatives much more often than one would expect from its population prevalence. Crohn's disease is more strongly familial than ulcerative colitis. The occurrence of both diseases in the same family is too frequent to be due to chance and implies a genetic and/or an environmental relationship between them.

The increasing incidence of Crohn's disease, in the past 50 years, cannot have been due to changes in the gene pool and must be due to a strong environmental cause of the disease. Yet, the familial pattern indicates that genetic factors are important. There has been no demonstration of the involvement of a major gene and a quantitative genetic basis to susceptibility to the environment is more likely.

The family studies raise the question of the entity of the two diagnoses and clinicians should not ignore the possibility that they are merely variants of the same disease process. The familial, epidemiological and clinical data could be due to their having a shared genetic basis, ulcerative colitis developing with a partial genotype and Crohn's disease with a fuller genotype, whilst two environmental factors are involved, one for inflammatory bowel disease and the other an additive factor for Crohn's disease.

References

1 Crohn, B. B.: The broadening concept of regional ileitis. Am. J. dig. Dis. *1:* 97–99 (1934).
2 Allchin, W. H.: Ulcerative colitis. Proc. R. Soc. Med. *2:* 59–63 (1909).
3 Kirsner, J. B.: Genetic aspects of inflammatory bowel disease. Clin. Gastroenterol. *2:* 557–575 (1973).
4 Sherlock, P.; Bell, B. M.; Steinberg, H.; Almy, T. P.: Familial occurrence of regional enteritis and ulcerative colitis. Gastroenterology *45:* 413–420 (1963).
5 Korelitz, B. I.: Epidemiological evidence for a hereditary component in Crohn's disease; in Peña, Weterman, Booth, Strober, Recent advances in Crohn's disease, pp. 208–212 (Martinus Nijhoff, The Hague 1981).
6 Farmer, R. G.; Michener, W. M.; Mortimer, E. A.: Studies of family history among patients with inflammatory bowel disease. Clin. Gastroenterol. *9:* 271–227 (1980).
7 Kemler, B. J.; Glass, D.; Alpert, E.: HLA studies of families with multiple cases of inflammatory bowel disease (IBD). Gastroenterology *78:* 1194 (1980).
8 Klein, G. L.; Ament, M. E.; Sparkes, R. S.: Monozygotic twins with Crohn's disease. A case report. Gastroenterology *79:* 931–933 (1980).
9 Morichau-Beauchant, M.; Matuchansky, C.; Dofing, J.-L.; Yver, L.; Morichau-Beauchant, J.: Entérite regionale chez des jumeaux homozygotes. Revue de la littérature à propos de lle cas rapporté. Gastroenterol. clin. biol. *1:* 783–788 (1977).
10 Mayberry, J. F.; Rhodes, J.; Newcombe, R. G.: Familial prevalence of inflammatory bowel disease in relatives of patients with Crohn's disease. Br. med. J. *i:* 84 (1980).
11 Whorwell, P. J.; Eade, O. E.; Hossenbocus, A.; Bamforth, J.: Crohn's disease in a husband and wife. Lancet *ii:* 186–187 (1978).
12 Zetzel, L.: Crohn's disease in a husband and wife. Lancet *ii:* 583 (1978).
13 Rosenberg, J. C.; Kraft, S. C.; Kirsner, J. B.: Inflammatory bowel disease in all three members of one family. Gastroenterology *70:* 759–760 (1976).

14 Paulley, J. W.: Ulcerative colitis. Gastroenterology *16:* 566–576 (1950).
15 Banks, B. M.; Korelitz, B. J.; Zetzel, L.: The course of nonspecific ulcerative colitis. Review of twenty years experience and late results. Gastroenterology *32:* 983–1012 (1957).
16 Kirsner, J. B.; Spencer, J. A.: Family occurrences of ulcerative colitis, regional enteritis and ileocolitis. Ann. intern. Med. *59:* 133–144 (1963).
17 Cowan, W. K.: Genetics of duodenal and gastric ulcer. Clin. Gastroenterol. *2:* 539–546 (1973).
18 Mallinson, C. N.; Candy, J. C.; Cowan, R.; Prior, A.: Two first degree relatives with dilatation of the colon due to Crohn's disease. Guys Hosp. Rep. *22:* 211–220 (1973).

Dr. R. B. McConnell, 2, Countisbury Drive, Liverpool L16 OJJ (UK)

Front. gastrointest. Res., vol. 11, pp. 12–16 (Karger, Basel 1986)

Familial Occurrence of Chronic Inflammatory Bowel Disease

I. R. Sanderson, S. K. F. Chong, J. A. Walker-Smith

Department of Child Health, St Bartholomew's Hospital,
West Smithfield, London, UK

Introduction

The first survey of the familial occurrence of chronic inflammatory bowel disease done over 20 years ago showed that 8% of patients had an affected family member [1]. *Singer* et al. [2] pointed out that surveys of this kind may be limited by patients being unaware of their relatives' illnesses. Families may be widely dispersed, and older relatives may no longer be living. Performing a survey on children with chronic inflammatory bowel disease, rather than adults, affords an opportunity to overcome this limitation as the majority of their first degree relatives will be living in the same household and most of their second degree relatives will still be alive.

Methods

A questionnaire was sent to the parents of 152 children attending the Paediatric Inflammatory Bowel Disease Clinic at St Bartholomew's Hospital. This asked for the name and address of any relative of their child who may have chronic inflammatory bowel disease. The relationship of the family and the type of inflammatory bowel disease was also requested.

All first-degree relatives in whom inflammatory bowel disease had been reported in the questionnaire were interviewed to check the diagnosis and biopsies, where available, were reviewed. If a second-degree relative was affected the child's parents were questioned about the diagnosis.

152 questionnaires were sent out of which 84 were returned within 3 weeks. Those who had not replied by that time were contacted by telephone and asked the questions directly. Fifteen parents were not traced. Three of the children were adopted.

Results

The children attending the clinic were diagnosed as having either Crohn's disease (91), ulcerative colitis (26) or indeterminate colitis (35) on clinical features, radiology, colonoscopy and multiple mucosal biopsies. One case of Behçet's colitis was included in the indeterminate colitis group.

For each group, the family members with chronic inflammatory bowel disease were recorded together with their diagnosis (table I–III).

The proportion of children that have a first-degree relative with chronic inflammatory bowel disease is similar for each of the three diseases (6–9%). However, whereas the children with *indeterminate* and *ulcerative colitis* have, in the main, relations with a type of disease similar to their own, those with *Crohn's disease* have relatives with all types of disease. 100% of the children with ulcerative colitis who had a family history were girls, compared to 66% of all 24 children with ulcerative colitis.

The occurrence of a first- or second-degree relative affected with chronic inflammatory bowel disease is high (16%). It occurs in 15% of children with Crohn's disease, 30% of those with ulcerative colitis, and 10% of those with indeterminate colitis.

Discussion

Overall, 16% of the 134 children with chronic inflammatory bowel disease in this study have a first- or second-degree relative with inflammatory bowel disease. This is at the lower end of the range of previous surveys reviewed by *Farmer* et al. [3]. The intermingling of ulcerative colitis and Crohn's disease in relatives suggests they may have related aetiologies. Such familial incidence has been attributed to genetically mediated mechanisms. However, contact transmission of an infectious agent or agents is not excluded by these observations. Spouses developing Crohn's disease have been described, albeit very exceptionally, in 8 cases in the world literature [4]. These findings are consistent with the concept of *McConnell* [5] which regards ulcerative colitis and Crohn's disease as prototypes of a single disease process with two polygenic systems determining liability possessing genes in common. Possession of a few of these genes predisposes to ulcerative colitis, whereas a more complete genotype predisposes to Crohn's disease. Nevertheless, environmental factors may be important. 9% of the 79 children with Crohn's disease have a first-degree relative with chronic inflammatory bowel disease. The same proportion was found in a study done on all age groups in Cardiff [6]. In

Table I. Crohn's disease (91 sent questionnaire, 40 replied (1 adopted), 40 contacted by telephone, 11 not traced)

Initials	Sex	First-degree relative	Second-degree relative	More distant relative
S.A.	M		maternal aunt (Crohn's disease)	
D.B.	F	father (UC)		
A.B.	F	mother (UC)		great aunt (UC)
B.B.	F		maternal aunt (UC)	
J.C.	F	mother (Crohn's disease)		maternal great uncle (UC)
G.D.	F			
J.H.	F		paternal uncle (Crohn's disease)	
K.H.	M		maternal grandmother (UC)	
G.H.	M		maternal grandmother (UC)	
P.I.	M	brother (Crohn's disease)[1]		
G.L.	M			maternal cousin (indeterminate colitis)
D.L.	M			paternal 2nd cousin (Crohn's disease)
D.W.	F	mother (UC)		
D.W.	M	mother (Crohn's disease)		
S.Y.	M	brother (indeterminate colitis)[1]		maternal 2nd cousin (Crohn's disease)

7/79 (9%) first-degree relative with chronic inflammatory bowel disease; 5/79 (6%) second-degree relative with chronic inflammatory bowel disease.

UC = Ulcerate colitis.

[1] Both brothers developed inflammatory bowel disease subsequent to diagnosis in sibling.

Table II. Ulcerative colitis (UC) (26 sent questionnaire, 24 replied (2 adopted), 1 contacted by telephone, 1 not traced)

Initials	Sex	First-degree relative	Second-degree relative	More distant relative
K. B.	F		paternal grandmother (UC)	
C. B.	F		paternal grandmother (UC)	
K. C.	F		paternal grandmother (UC)	
S. G.	F		Maternal uncle (colitis ?type)	
J. L.	F	mother (UC)	maternal grandmother (UC)	
M. M.	F		maternal aunt (Crohn's disease)	
H. M.	F	father (UC)		

2/23 (9%) first-degree relatives with chronic inflammatory bowel disease; 6/23 (26%) second-degree relatives with chronic inflammatory bowel disease.

Table III. Indeterminate colitis (35 sent questionnaire, 20 replied, 12 contacted by telephone, 3 not traced)

Initial	Sex	First-degree relative	Second-degree relative	More distant relative
H. B.	M	mother (indeterminate colitis)	maternal grandmother (colitis)	maternal great uncle (colitis)
J. J.	F			great great aunt (UC)
R. M.	F			cousin (UC)
A. T.	M		maternal grandfather (UC)	
A. Z.	M	sister (Behcet's colitis)		

2/32 (6%) first-degree relative with chronic inflammatory bowel disease; 2/32 (6%) second-degree relative with chronic inflammatory bowel disease.

UC = Ulcerative colitis.

that study, 11 of 13 of the affected first-degree relatives were siblings whereas in the present study, the majority (5 of 7) are parents. However, the number of siblings affected may increase in the future in a childhood population such as ours. For instance, were the study to be performed on the same cohort of children when they reach an age similar to those included in the Cardiff study, a higher proportion of children with affected first-degree relatives would be found. Indeed, had our study been performed at an earlier date, chronic inflammatory bowel disease would not yet have occurred in the 2 siblings recorded. If environmental factors are important in the aetiology of chronic inflammatory bowel disease, the difference between the two studies can be explained by the disease's rising incidence. It cannot be explained by a purely hereditary mechanism; for in inherited disease the ratio of people in one generation to those in another will not change with time except when there is a population shift of an evolutionary advantage to the affected person.

References

1   Kirsner, J. B.; Spencer, J. A.: Family occurrence of ulcerative colitis, regional ileitis and ileocolitis. Ann. intern. Med. *59:* 133–144 (1963).
2   Singer, H. C.; Anderson, J. G. D.; Frischer, H.; Kirsner, J. B.: Family aspects of inflammatory bowel disease. Gastroenterology *61:* 423–430 (1971).
3   Farmer, R. G.; Michener, W. M.; Mortimer, E. A.: Studies of family history among patients with inflammatory bowel disease. Clin. Gastroenterol. *9:* 271–278 (1980).
4   Kirsner, J. B.; Shorter, R. G.: Recent developments in non-specific inflammatory bowel disease. New Engl. J. Med. *306:* 837–848 (1982).
5   McConnell, R. B.: Inflammatory bowel disease: newer views of genetic influence, in Berk, Developments in digestive diseases, pp. 129–138, (Lea & Febiger, Philadelphia 1980).
6   Mayberry, J. F.; Rhodes, J.; Newcombe, R. G.: Family prevalence of inflammatory bowel disease in relatives of patients with Crohn's disease. Br. med. J. *280:* 84 (1980).

I. R. Sanderson, MD, Department of Child Health, St. Bartholomew's Hospital,
West Smithfield, London EC1 (UK)

Front. gastrointest. Res., vol. 11, pp. 17–26 (Karger, Basel 1986)

Association of Inflammatory Bowel Disease in Families

Richard G. Farmer[a], *William M. Michener*[b1]

[a] Division of Medicine, and [b] Division of Education, Cleveland Clinic Foundation, Cleveland, Ohio, USA

Although inflammatory bowel disease (IBD) has been known to occur in families for many years [1–3] the reports by *Kirsner and Spencer* [4] in 1963 and *Almy and Sherlock* [5] in 1966 stimulated a considerable amount of interest in this phenomenon. Subsequently, over the next 10 years, a number of other reports appeared [6–10]. A study from the University of Chicago in 1971 [8] described a familial occurrence rate of 17.5%, with 113 of 646 patients with IBD reporting positivity for a similar illness among various members of their families. It has been observed that IBD may occur in mulitple family members and a particular predilection was noted for familial aggregation of patients with ankylosing spondylitis in Crohn's disease [9–11]. However, no pattern has emerged which suggests a specific genetic link [12]. In a progress report in 1976, *Lewkonia and McConnell* [13] noted that study of the families of patients with IBD leaves no doubt that ulcerative colitis and Crohn's disease are closely associated. This association within families may be due to a common environmental etiology, but more probably it is due to a shared genetic background. A recent environmental review [14] further emphasized the complexity and apparent heterogeneity of the disease. The most recent association described in patients with IBD has been the possible relationship of familial occurrence of primary sclerosing cholangitis in association with ulcerative colitis [15].

Despite the increased interest in IBD and the increasing interest in familial, genetic, or environmental factors which might relate to the diseases, there is relatively little specificity concerning the significance of a positive family history for patients with IBD. Reasons for this have included the difficulty of interviewing a large number of patients using a similar technique and obtaining similar information. This problem was

[1] The authors wish to acknowledge *Susan Peppercorn* and *William Cusick* for their data collection.

addressed by *Singer* et al. [8] in which they were able to obtain data from 646 patients from an original group of 876. They noted that there were limitations to studies such as theirs and the limitations included: (1) the failure to obtain a 100% return on questionnaires; (2) the variation in detail of information provided by different probands; (3) the possible failure of a relative to report existing IBD because of a lack of awareness or a appropriate recognition of its presence, and (4) the inability to classify the bowel disease with 100% certainty in all cases.

In 1980 [16] we reported a study of family histories of 838 patients with onset of IBD before the age of 21. The purpose was to investigate the presence of IBD in additional family members, and all patients were interviewed and follow-up informtion was obtained from 826. Among 316 patients with ulcerative colitis, 93 (29%) had positive family histories for IBD. Among 522 patients with Crohn's disease, 187 (35%) had positive family histories for IBD. Those involved included 15% of immediate family members, including 6% of siblings of patients with ulcerative colitis and 7.5% of siblings with Crohn's disease. There were more than one family member found to have IBD in 21 instances of patients with ulcerative colitis (6.6%) and 46 instances (8.8%) of patients with Crohn's disease. Two families had 8 members afflicted and 3–5 members of families were involved 18 times. Thus, our study disclosed a positive family history for patients with IBD of about one-third overall and about 15% in the immediate family. The purpose of the current study was to update and expand this information using data from this cohort of patients with a longer follow-up time.

Methodology

From 1955 to 1974, there were 838 patients with IBD diagnosed at the Cleveland Clinic Foundation whose age of onset was 20 years or younger at the time of the diagnosis. Definite vertification of the diagnosis of ulcerative colitis or Crohn's disease was established by review of the clinical records, clinical and other diagnostic information, pathological and histological data, and observation of the clinical course of the patient during the follow-up period. For our record-keeping purposes, the diagnosis was considered to be established at the time the original diagnosis was made in our institution, regardless of whether a diagnosis of IBD had been entertained prior to the patient being seen at the Cleveland Clinic. Thus, there is a uniformity of record keeping, data collection and follow-up information. The latter was obtained by re-examination and/or re-interview of the patient.

The interview process was conducted by specifically trained personnel. The interviewers were often of similar age to the respondents, were sympathetic to their problems and questions, and spent adequate amounts of time obtaining the information. This technique was well received and facilitated cooperation by the patients. This technique has been used on an ongoing basis since 1973, and data is regularly updated.

Table I. Association of IBD in families

Patients[1]	Number of patients with positive family history	Mean duration of follow-up, years	Lost to follow up	Dead
Ulcerative colitis (n = 316)	93	17.8	10	4
Crohn's disease (n = 522)	187	16.7	15	10
Total (n = 838)	280		25	14

[1] Diagnosis made at Cleveland Clinic, 1955–1974.

Table II. Causes of death (14 patients)

Ulcerative colitis (n = 4)	Crohn's disease (n = 10)
Alcoholic cirrhosis 1 Cerebral aneurysm 1 Unknown 2	postoperative 3 myocarditis and pneumonia 1 carcinoma, small intestine 1 intestinal cancer, site unknown 1 drug overdose 1 auto accident 1 unknown 2

After verificationof the original diagnosis, it was established with the patient as to his or her knowledge of the nature of the diagnosis, definite knowledge of a similar diagnosis having been made among various family members, and verification of the number of siblings present in the immediate family. For purposes of this study, 'immediate family members' include parents and siblings. Additional family members include aunts, uncles and first-degree cousins in a blood line; although not made a part of this study, data concerning grandparents was also established.

The core data formed the basis of our 1980 publication [16]. The purpose of the current study was to ascertain whether or not additional family members had developed IBD among the group of families with positive family histories in the initial study.

Results

From January 1, 1955, to December 31, 1974, IBD was diagnosed in 838 patients 20 years old or younger at the time at the Cleveland Clinic. There were 316 patients with ulcerative colitis, 162 males and 154 females, and 522 patients with crohn's disease, 298 males and 224

Table III. Additional family members with IBD[1]

Original study[2] 838 patients Family history of IBD[2]	Ulcerative colitis 316 patients 93 patients (29%)				Crohn's disease 522 patients 187 patients (35%)			
	Original number[2]	New[1]	Total[1]	%	Original number[2]	New[1]	Total[1]	%
Parents	31	1	32	10.1	48	2	50	9.5
Siblings	19	4	23	7.2	39	4	43	8.2
Relatives[3]	43	10	53	16.7	100	12	112	21.3
Total	93	15	108	34	187	18	205	39
Grand total Original[2], 280 (34%) Subsequent[1], 313 (37.3%)								

[1] 1984.
[2] 1974.
[3] Aunts, uncles, first cousins – direct bloodline.

Table IV. Additional family members with IBD, immediate family[1]

Original study[2]	Ulcerative colitis				Crohn's disease			
838 patients Family history positive[2] Immediate family	316 patients 50 patients (15.8%)				522 patients 87 patients (16.6%)			
	Original number[2]	New[1]	Total[1]	%	Original number[2]	New[1]	Total[1]	%
Father-son	4	1	5	1.6	14	0	14	2.7
Father-daughter	8	0	8	2.5	6	1	7	1.3
Mother-son	10	0	10	3.2	14	1	15	2.9
Mother-daughter	9	0	9	2.8	14	1	15	2.9
Sibling-sibling	19	4	23	7.3	39	4	43	8.2
Total	50	5	55	17.4	87	7	94	18.0

Grand total
Original, 137 (16.3%)[2]
New, 12
New total, 149 (17.8%)[1]

[1] 1984.
[2] 1974.

females. The mean age at diagnosis was 15 years and the mean follow-up for patients with ulcerative colitis was 11.8 and 7.7 years for the patients with Crohn's disease (this latter phenomenon represented an increasing number of patients with Crohn's disease seen during the latter half of the study). Specific breakdown of the age distribution of the patients and the distribution during the half decades seen during this 20-year period are included in our previous report [16].

Among the 838 patients with IBD, 280 (34%) had family histories positive for IBD with at least 1 other members afflicted (table I). There were 93 patients with ulcerative colitis who had family histories positive for IBD (29%) and 187 with Crohn's disease who had family histories positive for IBD (35%). As noted in table I, by 1984, the follow-up history had been updated to a mean of 17.8 years for the patients with ulcerative colitis, and a mean of 16.7 years for the patients with Crohn's disease. There have been 25 patients lost to follow-up during this entire period of time and 14 patients have died. The causes of death are listed in table II.

Among the 280 patients with a positive family history for IBD at the time of the original study [16], there were 680 siblings (in the 280 families) for a mean of 2.4 siblings in the affected families. In the 558 without a positive family history, 1,205 siblings were present, a mean of 2.2 siblings per family. The purpose of the study was to focus on the 280 patients with a positive family history to determine whether or not additional family members had developed IBD since the close of the original study in December, 1974. There were 33 additional family members of these 280 patients who had developed IBD during the subsequent follow-up period (table III). This included 3 parents, 8 siblings and 22 other close relatives. As can be noted in table III, there was a slight preponderence for positive family history among patient with Crohn's disease with an overall percentage of 39% involvement. At the time of the initial study [16] there were 13 patients with ulcerative colitis who had a positive family history affecting a grandparent; subsequently, there have been two additional grandparents who have become afflicted (total of 4.7%). There were 29 patients with Crohn's disease with a positive family history for grandparents and there have been three additional (total of 6%). However, data involving grandparents is not as precise as those involving other family members and is not included.

Of particular concern are those immeditate family members who develop IBD subsequent to the index case. As noted in table IV, there were 50 patients (15.8%) with ulcerative colitis who had a positive immediate family history; there were 87 patients with Crohn's disease (16.6%) with a positive immediate family history. Subsequently, 5 further patients with ulcerative colitis have been identified in the immediate

Table V. Multiple members of family with IBD

	Ulcerative colitis		Crohn's disease	
	n	%	n	%
Original study[1]	21/316	6.6	46/522	8.8
Subsequent study[2]	28/316	8.9	51/522	9.8

[1] 1974.
[2] 1984.

family (4 siblings) and 7 immediate family members with Crohn's disease (4 siblings). In no case was the parent/child involvement higher than 3.2% in any of the specific categories encountered. The overall incidence of immediate family member involvement is 17.8%.

In the initial study [16] there were 21 instances of multiple members of family involvement (three or more) for patients with ulcerative colitis (6.6%) and 46 instances (8.8%) of Crohn's disease. Subsequently, there are now 28 families with more than three members with ulcerative colitis (8.9%) and 51 families with three or more members involved with Crohn's disease (9.8%) (table V).

In addition to the concern over family member involvement with IBD, another worry to patients is the potential for development of cancer of the digestive system. Thus, this study focused on specific instances of cancer occurring in the families of these patients. There were three family members without IBD who developed colorectal cancer (uncle, grandmother, grandfather) and one grandfather without IBD who developed stomach cancer. One grandfather with ulcerative colitis developed cancer of the stomach and other grandfather with probable Crohn's disease developed cancer of the rectum. An uncle with Crohn's disease developed cancer of the stomach; other than these cases, there were no instances of gastrointestinal malignancy reported.

Another concern is the development of IBD in other nonbloodline family members with IBD. One patient whose ulcerative colitis was diagnosed in the early 1960s has a husband who subsequently also developed ulcerative colitis. A second man whose diagnosis of ulcerative colitis was in the early 1970s has a wife who subsequently developed ulcerative colitis, and a third man, with Crohn's disease, has a wife who developed ulcerative colitis. In addition, 1 half-brother was identified with ulcerative colitis, 1 second cousin with ulcerative colitis, 1 third cousin with ulcerative colitis, and 1 great aunt with Crohn's disease were identified among patients in this group of 280 with IBD.

Discussion

Prior to our 1980 report [16], the 1971 University of Chicago [8] report of a 17.5% familial occurrence rate was the highest reported in the literature. Subsequently, *Korelitz* [17] reported a 20% incidence of positive family history among patients with Crohn's disease. Previous studies [4,5] had indicated that the probability of a familial occurrence due to chance alone was not great and that there must be a genetic factor present. Further, it appeared that the familial incidence was increasing compared with the 1950 Mayo Clinic Study [2] in which a positive family history was found in only 1.3%. Interest in various subsets of the IBD population included a specific look at Jewish patients [8] and those with Crohn's disease and ankylosing spondylists [9–11]. However, no specific genetic pattern emerged and reviews [12, 13] have emphasized that 'ulcerative colitis and Crohn's disease are closely associated' and that the association within families 'may be due to a common environmental etiology but more likely it is due to a shared genetic background" [13]. Further, distribution of IBD has been found to be both 'vertical' (from one generation to another) and 'horizontal' (multiple members in the same generation) so that the question of multiple genes with low penetrance, and/or a shared genetic background with added environmental factors, remains unclear.

Our study in 1980 documented the occurrence of IBD in approximately one-third of the families of those patients whose illness began in childhood or adolescence [16]. In the current study, the mean follow-up for ulcerative colitis patients has been increased by 6 years and the mean follow-up for patients with Crohn's disease has been increased by 9 years. This has led to a 5% increase in the number of famly members afflicted with IBD. However, the predominant family members afflicted continue to be siblings and first cousins (the 'horizontal' pattern) rather than occurring from generation to generation. Further, there has been a considerable increase in sophistication and understanding by patients and their families as to the nature of IBD in recent years, so that the diagnosis of additional family members may be facilitated by this process. Nonetheless, the association of a positive family history in over one-third of patients with childhood onset IBD makes this an important clinical phenomenon and one of which the treating physician must be aware. There are many problems peculiar to the child or adolescent with Crohn's disease [18] or ulcerative colitis [19] and we have reviewed and compared the clinical course of these two diseases with childhood onset [20]. There are many factors which create problems for families with a child or adolescent with inflammatory bowel disease, and the fear of the disease occurring in additional family members only accentuates this anxiety. Although 'markers' have been sought, such as HLA-B27 [11] the infrequency of this finding and the lack of specificity of other diagnostic features has not helped this dilemma. As has also been noted, a relative lack of specificity of factors, including 'genetic, environmental, or both' [13] has likewise not given any more specific clues other than the observation of clustering in families. Therefore, the significance of this current work is that an impressively high number (over one-third) of patients whose onset of IBD in childhood or adolescence will subsequently have additional family members affected. However, this increase does not progress in a linear fashion over time. There was a 5% increase in the number of patients afflicted with IBD during the additional follow-up period (a mean value of 6–9 years), but there was not a substantial parent/child relationship to the disease pattern. Thus, our data suggests that while genetic factors may undoubtedly increase susceptibility, that environmental and other factors may also be present, and there is no specific genetic pattern identified which would indicate that family counseling with avoidance of childbearing should be suggested for patients with inflammatory bowel disease.

References

1   Jackman, R. J.; Bargen, J. A.: Familial occurrence of chronic ulcerative colitis (thrombo-ulcerative colitis): report of cases. Am. J. dig. Dis. 9: 147–149 (1942).

2   Sloan, W. P., Jr.; Bargen J. A.; Gage, R. P.: Life histories of patients with chronic ulcerative colitis: a review of 2,000 cases. Gastroenterology 16: 25 (1950).

3   Felsen, J.; Wolarsky, W.: Familial incidence of ulcerative colitis and ileitis. Gastroenterology 28: 412–417 (1955).

4   Kirsner, J. B.; Spencer, J. A.: Family occurrences of ulcerative colitis, regional enteritis, and ileocolitis. Ann. intern. Med. 59: 133–144 (1963).

5   Almy, T. P.; Sherlock, P.: Genetic aspects of ulcerative colitis and regional enteritis. Gastroenterology 51: 757–763 (1966).

6   Barker, W. F.: Familial history of patients with ulcerative colitis. Am. J. Surg. 103: 25–26 (1962).

7   Binder, V.; Weeke, E.; Olsen, J. H.; Anthonisen, P.; Riis, P.: A genetic study of ulcerative colitis. Scand. J. Gastroent. 1: 49–56 (1966).

8   Singer, M. C.; Anderson, J. G. D.; Frischer, H.; Kirsner, J. B.: Familial aspects of inflammatory bowel disease. Gastroenterology 61: 423–430 (1971).

9   Kuspira, J.; Bhambhani, R.; Singh, S. M.; Links, H.: Familial occurrence of Crohn's disease. Hum. Hered. 22: 239–242 (1972).

10 Dassei, P. M.: A familial pattern in inflammatory disease of the bowel (Crohn's disease and ulcerative colitis). Dis. Colon Rectum 20: 699–701 (1977).

11 Macrae, I.; Wright, V.: A family study of ulcerative colitis. With particular reference to ankylosing spondylitis and sacroilitis. Ann. rheum. Dis. 32: 16–20 (1973).

12 Kirsner, J. B.: Genetic aspects of inflammatory bowel disease. Clin. Gastroenterol. *2:* 557–575 (1973).
13 Lewkonia, R. M.; McConnel, R. B.: Familial inflammatory bowel disease—heredity or environment? Gut *17:* 235–243 (1976).
14 Mayberry, J. F.; Rhodes, J.: Epidemiological aspects of Crohn's disease. A review of the literature. Gut *25:* 886–899 (1984).
15 Quigley, E. M. M.; LaRusso, N. F.; Ludwig, J.; MacSween, R. N. M.; Birnie G. G.; Watkinson, G.: Familial occurrence of primary sclerosing cholangitis and ulcerative colitis. Gastroenterology *85:* 1160–1165 (1983).
16 Farmer, R. G.; Michener, W. M.; Mortimer, E. A.: Studies of family history among patients with inflammatory bowel disease. Clin. Gastroenterol. *9:* 271–278 (1980).
17 Korelitz, B. I.: Epidemiological and psychosocial aspects of inflammatory bowel disease with observations on children, families, and pregnancy. Am. J. Gastroent. *77:* 929–933 (1982).
18 Michener, W. M.; Farmer, R. G.; Mortimer, E. A.: Long term prognosis of ulcerative colitis with onset in childhood or adolescence. J. clin. Gastroent. *1:* 301–305 (1979).
19 Farmer, R. G.; Michener, W. M.: Prognosis of Crohn's disease with onset in childhood or adolescence. Dig. Dis. Sci. *24:* 752–757 (1979).
20 Michener, W. M.; Greenstreet, R. L.; Farmer, R. G.: Comparison of the clinical features of Crohn's disease and ulcerative colitis with onset in childhood or adolescence. Cleve. Clin. Q. *49:* 13–16 (1982).

Richard G. Farmer, MD, Cleveland Clinic Foundation, 9500 Euclid Avenue, Cleveland, OH 44106 (USA)

Front. gastrointest. Res., vol. 11, pp. 27–34 (Karger, Basel 1986)

Prevalence of Crohn's Disease in First-Degree Relatives of Patients with Crohn's Disease

Irene T. Weterman, A. S. Peña

Department of Gastroenterology, University Hospital, Leiden, The Netherlands

Introduction

We recently reported a detailed family study of 400 unrelated Dutch patients with Crohn's disease (CD) in 8% of whom we found a second case of CD among first-degree relatives [1]. The present report concerns the subsequent occurrence of Crohn's disease in first-degree relatives of these and new patients attending our department. To assess similarity in these features as an indication of a hereditary predisposition, we also analysed the clinical patterns and the histopathological features of the disease in eight families with two or more siblings suffering from CD.

Materials and Methods

Among 400 unrelated Dutch patients already reported, one new case of a first-degree relative, a 13-year-old son of a father with CD, occurred in the last 2 years. During this period the family history of 46 new CD patients attending our department was obtained in the same way as for the first group and the diagnosis was reached on the basis of the same clinical, radiological, endoscopic, and/or histopathologic criteria [1]. Two new families with a first-degree relative with CD were identified, one being the youngest sister of a female patient and the other the father of a male patient.

Results

Among the total group of 446 unrelated Dutch patients a first-degree relative with CD was found in 35 families, which means a prevalence of 7.9%. The family relationships were distributed as follows: father-son, 3 pairs; father-daughter, 8 pairs; mother-son, 1 pair; mother-daughter, 1

Table I. Prevalence of Crohn's disease (CD) in first-degree relatives of patients with CD
(n = 446; hospital population)

Family relationship	CD	%	Prevalence (10^5)
Father (n = 446)	8	1.8	1,794
Mother (n = 446)	1	0.2	224
Brother (n = 735)	11	1.5	1,497
Sister (n = 700)	13	1.9	1,857
Son (n = 300)	1	0.3	333
Daughter (n = 283)	3	1.1	1,060
Total (n = 2,910)	37	1.2	1,237

pair; and brother-sister, 24 pairs. Two families each had 3 siblings suffering from CD, and we found 1 monozygotic twin with CD. Table I shows the prevalence of CD among the first-degree relatives.

In eight families with more than 1 child with CD, both the propositus and the affected relative are being followed-up in our department. Table II shows the age and year of onset, the localization of the disease at the time of referral to our department, the presence or absence of granuloma in resected tissue or biopsy samples, and the degree of sharing of HLA haplotypes of the Crohn's–Crohn's sibling pairs.

Discussion

It is interesting to note that even though the present study was not a true epidemiological one in that it was based on a population of patients attending the Leiden University Hospital, the prevalence of CD in first-degree relatives is similar to that found by *Mayberry* et al. [2] in a formal epidemiological study. In patients residing in Cardiff these authors found 7 siblings suffering from CD in a total of 437 siblings, giving a prevalence of 1,602/10^5. Our calculations yielded a prevalence of 1,672/10^5, based on 24 affected siblings in a study population of 1,435. If the prevalence of CD in The Netherlands is similar to that in the population of Cardiff, i.e. 56/10^5, or Copenhagen [3], i.e. 32/10^5, Crohn's disease may be 30–50 times more common in siblings than in the general population.

We mentioned elsewhere [1] that the prevalence between siblings and children was almost significant, and that this probably indicated that the children had not been alive long enough to develop the disease. This conclusion has been now confirmed by the results of a further 2-year follow-up study where we found that a 13-year-old son of one of our patients had developed CD.

It can be seen in table II that in 6 affected sib-pairs the onset of the disease occurred 1–5 years apart, the difference in time suggesting that environmental factors are important for the expression of the disease. The 2 affected sib-pairs, with more than 10 years difference in the time of onset, point to a genetic predisposition. There appears to be more affected sib-pairs with shortest difference in onset of disease than those with more than 10 years difference, suggesting that environmental factor(s) are more important than genetic factors.

According to *Morichau-Beauchant* et al. [30], the importance of genetic factors can be assessed best in identical twins. In 9 out of 10 twin pairs discussed by these authors, the age at diagnosis and the localization were very similar. Five of the 8 sib-pairs developed the disease at about the same age, whereas in the other 3 the difference in the age of onset was between 10 and 23 years.

Since a similar clinical pattern and identical pathology seem to support a strong hereditary predisposition, we analysed these features in siblings of families with multiple cases of CD attending our department. As table II shows, the degree of similarity does not differ greatly from that observed in unrelated cases with CD.

It is worth mentioning that even the presence of granulomas may vary among first-degree relatives. In one sibling pair, granulomas (table II, No. 2) were found in biopsy specimens taken during endoscopy but no granulomas were found in the affected brother, who required more than one resection. In two other pairs the affected relative has not received surgical treatment and therefore it is not known with certainty whether they have granulomas. The HLA haplotype sharing, found between these Crohn's–Crohn's pairs, does not differ from the pattern seen with normal Mendelian segregation. Although the literature offers examples of similar clinical and chronological courses of the disease and identical pathology of the bowel, for example the 2 brothers reported by *Gelfand and Krone* [4], our observations point in the direction of environmental conditions as the decisive factors in the etiology of Crohn's disease. However, as *McConnell* [5] has stated, it is very unlikely that 3 or more members of one family would suffer from a disease solely due to environmental factors without other cases occurring in unrelated neighbors. Our series includes 2 families with 3 affected children, and in the medical literature we

Table II. Crohn's disease: family relationship, sex, year of onset, age at onset of the disease, localization, at time of referral, presence or absence of granuloma, and HLA haplotype sharing in Crohn's-Crohn's sibling pairs

Subject	Sex	Year of onset	Age at onset, years	Localization			Granuloma	Number of pairs sharing		
				ileum	ileum + colon	colon		2 haplotypes	1 haplotype	none
1	M	1965	24	+			+	+		
2	M¹	1962	21	+			+ (n.o.)	n.d.		
1	M	1978	39			+	+ (n.o.)			
2	M	1954	16		+		−			
1	F	1982	22	+			− (n.o.)	+		
3	F	1978	10.5		+		−			
1	F	1966	17	+			+		+	
3	F	1965	15			+	−			
1	F	1966	32		+		− (n.o.)		+	
2	M	1952	19	+			+			
1	M	1967	18	+			+		+	
3	F	1962	18	+			+			
1	M	1977	14	+			− (n.o.)			
3	F	1979	13		+		+	+		
1	M	1969	29	+			+			+
3	F	1971	29	+			+			

n.d. = Not done; n.o. = no operation;
1 = propositus; 2 = brother; 3 = sister.
¹ Identical twin.

Table III. Reported families with more than two siblings with Crohn's disease

Authors	Year	Number of families	Number of siblings
Brown and Scheiffly [10]	1939	1	3
Bargen (quoted by *Kirsner* [11])	1962	1	5
Almy and Sherlock [12]	1966	5	3 or more
Gelfand and Krone [4]	1970	1	3 and mother
Singer et al. [13]	1971	2	more than 2
Russe (quoted by *Kirsner* [11])	1972	1	5
Kuspira et al. [14]	1972	1	3
Strik and Strik [15]	1972	1	4
Mörl et al. [16]	1976	1	3
Korelitz [17]	1981	19	3 or more
Farmer et al. [18]	1981	15	3 or more
Achord et al. [19]	1982	1	5
Weterman and Peña [1]	1984	2	3
Total		51	

found 49 additional families with more than 2 affected siblings (table III). In a large case-controlled study performed in Britain, no evidence of time-space clustering was obtained [6] and, to the best of our knowledge, there is only one report of a small aggregation of unrelated patients with CD, which was found in a Cotswold village in England [7].

Two other observations also support a genetic predisposition for CD. One is the occurrence of CD in members of three generations, and three such families have been reported [8, 9, 17]. The other is a high degree of concordance in monozygotic twins and a low degree of concordance in dizygotic twins. The evidence published so far, which is summarized in table IV, amounts to 85% (17 out of 20) vs. 17% (1 out of 6) as it stands. Obviously, the sample error due to under-reporting may be large, and the present data should serve to encourage the recording of such cases, since it cannot offer a basis for firm conclusions. It is almost certain that discordant dizygotic twins are usually not described.

The segregation of the disease in first-degree relatives supports a multifactorial form of inheritance. At present, we do not know the exact prevalence of the disease in The Netherlands and therefore no definite risk estimates for CD can be made for this country.

Table IV. Published cases of twins with Crohn's disease

Concordant			Discordant		
Authors	year	number of twin pairs	authors	year	number of twin pairs
Monozygotic twins			Monozygotic twins		
Edwards [20]	1954	1	Anfanger [34]	1955	1
Freysz et al. [21]	1958	1	Lagercrantz [35]	1976	1
Niederlé [22]	1961	1	Weterman and Peña [1]	1984	1
Crismer et al. [23]	1963	1			
Janowitz (in Sherlock et al. [24])	1963	1			
Farago [25]	1967	1			
Hislop and Grant [26]	1969	1			
Milton-Thomson and Lennard-Jones [27]	1971	1			
Berg and Dencker [28]	1972	1			
Goldstein et al. [29]	1976	1			
Morichau-Beauchant et al. [30]	1977	1			
Carlisle and Hersh [31]	1978	1			
Hellers [32]	1979	3			
Klein et al. [33]	1980	1			
Weterman and Peña [1]	1984	1			
Total		17			
Dizygotic twins			Dizygotic twins		
Strik and Strik [15]	1972	1	Weterman and Peña [1]	1984	5

References

1 Weterman, I. T.; Peña, A. S.: Familial incidence of Crohn's disease in The Netherlands and a review of the literature. Gastroenterology *86:* 449–452 (1984).
2 Mayberry, J. F.; Rhodes, J.; Newcombe, R. G.: Familial prevalence of inflammatory bowel disease in relatives of patients with Corhn's disease. Br. med. J. *1:* 84 (1980).
3 Binder, V.; Both, H.; Hansen, P. K.; Hendriksen, C.; Kreiner, S.; Torp-Pedersen, K.: Incidence and prevalence of ulcerative colitis and Crohn's disease in the County of Copenhagen, 1962 to 1978. Gastroenterology *83:* 563–568 (1982).
4 Gelfand, M. D.; Krone, C. L.: Inflammatory bowel disease in a family. Observations related to pathogenesis. Ann. intern. Med. *72:* 903–907 (1970).
5 McConnell, R. B.: Genetic factors in Crohn's disease; in Engel, Larsson, Skandia International Symposia. Regional enteritis (Crohn's disease), pp. 220–230 (Nordiska/Bokhandelns Förlag, Stockholm 1971).
6 Miller, D. S.; Keighley, A.; Smith, P. G.; Hughes, A. O.; Langman, M. J. S.: A case-control method for seeking evidence of contagion in Crohn's disease. Gastroenterology *71:* 385–387 (1976).
7 Allan, R. N.; Ibbertson, G.; Pease, P. I.; Mackintosh, P.: Clustering of Crohn's disease in a Cotswold Village (Abstract). Q. J. Med. (in press).
8 Lifton, L. J.; Stafford, J. M.: Crohn's disease affecting three generations. Case reports and genetic typing. Am. J. Gastroent. *78:* 159–161 (1983).
9 Davis, P.: Quantitative sacroiliac scintigraphy in ankylosing spondylitis and Crohn's disease. A single family study. Ann. rheum. Dis. *38:* 241–243 (1979).
10 Brown, P. W.; Scheiffley, C.: Chronic regional enteritis occurring in three siblings. Am. J. dig. Dis. *6:* 257–261 (1939).
11 Kirsner, J. B.: Genetic aspects of inflammatory bowel disease. Clin. Gastroenterol. *2:* 557–575 (1973).
12 Almy, T. P.; Sherlock, P.: Genetic aspects of ulcerative colitis and regional enteritis. Gastroenterology *51:* 757–761 (1966).
13 Singer, H. C.; Anderson, J. G. D.; Frischer, H.; Kirsner, J. B.: Familial aspects of inflammatory bowel disease. Gastroenterology *61:* 423–430 (1971).
14 Kuspira, J.; Bhambhani, R.; Singh, S. M.; Links, H.: Familial occurrence of Crohn's disease. Hum. Hered. *22:* 239–242 (1972).
15 Strik, W. O.; Strik, W.: Familiares Auftreten der Enteritis Regionales bei zweieiigen Zwillingen und 2 weiteren Geschwistern. Münch. med. Wschr. *114:* 1852–1856 (1972).
16 Mörl, M.; Koch, H.; Rösch, W.; Frühmorgen, P.; Zeus, J.: Familiäre Enterocolitis regionalis Crohn. Dt. med. Wschr. *101:* 493–496 (1976).
17 Korelitz, B. I.: Epidemiological evidence for a hereditary component in Crohn's disease; in Peña, Weterman, Booth, Strober, Recent advances in Crohn's disease, developments in gastroenterology, vol. I, pp. 208–212 (Martinus Nijhoff, The Hague 1981).
18 Farmer, R. G.; Michener, W. M.; Sivak, D. S.: Studies of family history in inflammatory bowel disease; in Peña, Weterman, Booth, Strober, Recent Advances in Crohn's disease, developments in gastroenterology, vol. I, pp. 213–218 (Martinus Nijhoff, The Hague 1981).
19 Achord, J. L.; Gunn, H. C.; Jackson, J. F.: Regional enteritis and HLA concordance in multiple siblings. Dig. Dis. Sci. *27:* 330–332 (1982).
20 Edwards, H. C.: Crohn's disease; in Edwards, Recent advances in surgery; 4th ed., pp. 170–171 (Churchill, London 1954).

21 Freysz, H.; Haemmerli, A.; Kartagener, M.: Ileitis regionalis bei einem weiblichem Zwillingspaar. Gastroenterologia *89:* 75–82 (1958).
22 Niederlé, M. B.: Iléite régionale chez des jumelles univitellines. Archs Mal. Appar. dig. Mal. Nutr. *50:* 1245–1246 (1961).
23 Crismer, R.; Drèze, C.; Dodinval, P.: Maladie de Crohn a localisation iléo-caecale chez des jumeaux univitellins. Archs Mal. Appar. dig. Mal. Nutr. *52:* 957–969 (1963).
24 Sherlock, P.; Bell, B. M.; Steinberg, H.; Almy, T. P.: Familial occurrence of regional enteritis and ulcerative colitis. Gastroenterology *45:* 413–420 (1963).
25 Farago, E.: Enteritis regionales elofordulasa. Testvere. ornosi Hetilap. *108:* 1993–1994 (1967).
26 Hislop, I. G.; Grant, A. K.: Genetic tendency in Crohn's disease. Gut *10:* 994–995 (1969).
27 Milton-Thompson, G. J.; Lennard-Jones, J. E.: A pair of probable monozygotic twins with colonic Crohn's disease. Proc. R. Soc. Med. *64:* 570 (1971).
28 Berg, N. O.; Dencker, H.: Crohn's disease in monozygotic twins. Acta chir. scand. *138:* 633–635 (1972).
29 Goldstein, F.; Abraham, A. A.; Abramson, J.; Thornton, J. J.: Ileojejunitis in a pair of identical twins. Gastroenterology *71:* 670–674 (1976).
30 Morichau-Beauchant, M.; Matuchansky, C.; Dofing, J. L.; Yver, L.; Morichau-Beauchant, J.: Entérite régionale chez des jumeaux homozygotes. Revue de la litérature à propos du 11e cas rapporté. Gastroentérol. clin. biol. *1:* 763–788 (1977).
31 Carlisle, W. R.; Hersh, T.: Clinical manifestations of familial inflammatory bowel disease (IBD). Gastroenterology *74:* 1017A (1978).
32 Hellers, G.: Crohn's disease in Stockholm County 1955–1974. A study of epidemiology, results of Surgical treatment and long-term prognosis. Acta chir. scand., suppl *490* (1979).
33 Klein, G. L.; Ament, M. E.; Sparkes, R. S.: Monozygotic twins with Crohn's disease. A case report. Gastroenterology *79:* 931–933 (1980).
34 Anfanger, H.: Regional ileitis in children. Mount Sinai J. Med. *22:* 187–191 (1955).
35 Lagercrantz, R.: Crohn's disease in children and adolescents; in Weterman, Peña, Booth, The management of Crohn's disease, pp. 37–40 (Excerpta Medica, Amsterdam 1976).

Irene T. Weterman, MD, Department of Gastroenterology, University Hospital, Rijnsburgerweg 10, NL-2333 AA Leiden (The Netherlands)

Front. gastrointest. Res., vol. 11, pp. 35–41 (Karger, Basel 1986)

Tissue Antigens and Inflammatory Bowel Disease

A. Ellis, J. McKay, J. C. Woodrow, R. B. McConnell

The Gastroenterology Units of Broadgreen Hospital, Liverpool and the Royal Liverpool Hospital, and the Department of Medicine, University of Liverpool, UK

Both Crohn's disease and ulcerative colitis are *familial* diseases, approximately 10–30% of first-degree relatives of patients with either condition may also be affected [1, 2]. The lack of a simple mendelian inheritance pattern has been interpreted as indicating a polygenic mode of inheritance [3]. However, simply because a disease shows familial aggregation it does not necessarily follow that genetic factors are involved. Environmental influences may just as easily be the explanation. Another way of elucidating the importance of *genetic* factors in the aetiology of a disorder is to demonstrate an association between the disorder and an inherited marker trait. *Human leucocyte antigens* (HLA) were an obvious choice to study because of the multiple immune abnormalities which have been recorded in both patients [4, 5] with inflammatory bowel disease (IBD) and their close relatives [6].

Reports of HLA-IBD Associations

There have been numerous reports of the frequency of *HLA-A and HLA-B antigens* in both ulcerative colitis and Crohn's disease (table I). In the majority of studies there has been no difference in the frequencies of the various antigens between patients and control groups, or the significance was lost when corrected for the number of antigens tested. Even when significant differences were found there was no consistent pattern, overall, in the results from different centres for the same disease.

There have been fewer studies of *HLA-DR antigens* in inflammatory bowel disease (table II). Only in a study on ulcerative colitis from Japan was there a significant increase in an antigen (DR2) compared to controls [29]. All the other studies showed little difference in the frequencies of HLA-DR antigens between patient and control groups.

Table I. HLA-A and B antigens in inflammatory bowel disease

Study	Crohn's disease		Ulcerative colitis	
	number of patients	HLA association	number of patients	HLA association
Thorsby and Lie [7]	19	nil	–	–
Gleeson et al. [8]	18	nil	16	nil
Asquith et al. [9]	56	↓ (A9)	48	↑ (A11, B7)
Brewerton et al. [10]	–	–	30	nil
Jacoby and Jayson [11]	74	nil	–	–
Korsmeyer et al. [12]	8	nil	37	nil
Lewkonia et al. [13]	30	nil	–	nil
Russell et al. [14]	77	nil	51	nil
Bergman et al. [15]	62	↑ (A1, B14, B17)	100	nil
Mallas et al. [16]	100	nil	30	↑ (A2, BW35, BW40) (A10)
Nahir et al. [17]	–	–	44	↑ B5
Tsuchiya et al. [18]	–	–	58	↑ All ↓ (B7)
Berg-Loonen et al. [19]	51	↑ B18 ↓ (B5)	51	nil
Woodrow et al. [20]	43	nil	36	nil
Mowbray et al. [20]	–	–	60	↑ B5 ↓ (B7)
Hiwatashi et al. [21]	10	–	60	↑ (AW24) BW35
Delpre et al. [22]	18	nil	–	–
Eade et al. [23]	64	nil	–	–
Schwartz et al. [24]	22	nil	–	–
Peña et al. [25]	149	↑ (B14, B18) ↓ (A1, B8, BW35)	–	–
Burnham et al. [26]	67	nil	75	nil
Cohen et al. [27]	48	nil	–	–
Smolen et al. [28]	27	B12	30	nil
Asakura et al. [29]	–	–	40	↑ (AW24, BW52) ↓ (A11)

↑ = Antigen increased in frequency; ↓ = antigen decreased in frequency.
( ) corrected p not significant.

Table II. HLA-DR antigens in inflammatory bowel disease

Study	Crohn's disease		Ulcerative colitis	
	number of patients	HLA association	number of patients	HLA association
Peña et al. [25]	65	nil	–	–
Burnham et al. [26]	67	nil	75	nil
Cohen et al. [27]	47	nil	–	–
Smolen et al. [28]	27	nil	30	nil
Asakura et al. [29]	–	–	40	DR2
Ellis et al. [unpubl.]	63	nil	39	nil

Possible Reasons for Lack of HLA Association with IBD

It seems incomprehensible that diseases like Crohn's disease and ulcerative colitis, which have numerous immunological features, should not have an association with the major histocompatibility complex whereas coeliac disease for instance does. There may be several reasons for this.

(1) Failure to demonstrate a genuine association.

(a) Inadequate *numbers:* Many of the studies have been made on small numbers of controls and even smaller numbers of patients and this can lead to the so-called type II error.

(b) Poor selection of *controls:* Data on HLA antigen frequencies in control groups are often collated rather cursorily without attempting to match patient and control groups in any way. Frequently, the controls are not positively vetted to exclude the condition which is being studied. These oversights can cancel genuine and significant associations.

(c) *Technical* problems with reagents: These have been largely overcome by the use of internationally defined antisera through the histocompatibility workshops. It is now recognised that many of the antisera used in early studies were not homogeneous and have subsequently been split into two or more separate determinants. The association may be with only one of these determinants and not all of them, and therefore may be obscured if an antiserum which cannot distinguish the various determinants is used. An example of this type of association is that of Behçet's syndrome and HLA-B5. When B5 was shown to be a mixture of two separate determinants BW51 and 52 it was subsequently shown that the association was with BW51 alone [30].

(2) Heterogeneous patient material.

(a) *Diagnostic* criteria: When an individual patient has evidence of small bowel disease, fistulae or gross perianal involvement, the distinction from ulcerative colitis can be relatively easy. However, when the colon is the only organ affected the differentiation can be much more difficult. Evidence of transmural inflammation characteristic of Crohn's disease is not easily obtained without recourse to surgery. Macroscopically, predominantly right-sided lesions, skip areas and punctate lesions are helpful in diagnosing Crohn's disease; whilst microscopically focal non-specific inflammation and granulomata are useful. However, granulomata are only present in 60–70% of cases of Crohn's colitis [31]. Furthermore, about 10% of cases of idiopathic inflammatory bowel disease cannot be classified as one or the other, the so-called indeterminate colitis [32]. Thus, if a proportion of patients were to be assigned to the wrong disease group, this would have the effect of concealing any true association.

(b) Different associations with different *ethnic* populations: It has been shown in Graves' disease that in caucasian populations there is a significant association with HLA-DR3 but in the Japanese, amongst whom DR3 is very rare, there is an association instead with BW35 [33, 34]. Thus, if the three Japanese studies [18, 21, 29] are analysed together by the method of *Woolf* [35] and *Haldane* [36], a strong association is found between ulcerative colitis and HLA-B5/BW52 ($\chi^2 = 25.7$, $p < 0.0001$, combined relative risk 2.83). A similar analysis of the two Jewish studies on ulcerative colitis [17, 22] reveals significant associations with A10 ($\chi^2 = 13.9$, $p < 0.001$) and BW35 ($\chi^2 = 14.8$, $p < 0.001$). Analysis of the studies on caucasian populations [8, 10, 16, 19, 20, 26, 28] either failed to show an association with a particular antigen or there was significant heterogeneity in the results from different centres.

(c) An association between a disease and a genetic marker such as HLA may also be obscured by the fact that even within a well-defined patient group the association is not with all patients but with a certain *subgroup:* For example, the association between psoriasis and HLA-CW6 is between psoriasis vulgaris and not pustular psoriasis [37]. Attempts to correlate various parameters in Crohn's disease such as age of onset, site of disease, disease severity and sex have been unsuccessful [25].

Analysis of Our Results

We analysed our results on 63 patients with *Crohn's disease*, of whom 41 were granuloma positive and 16 were granuloma negative. HLA-B8 was more frequent in the granuloma-positive patients (19.5%) than the granuloma-negative patients (6.3%) and an even more obvious trend was seen with DR3 which was present in 39 and 19%, respectively. The reverse was true for DR2 which was less frequent in the granuloma-positive (17%) than in the granuloma-negative group (36%).

In *ulcerative colitis Asakura* et al. [29] showed that DR2 was more strongly associated with total colitis (73%) than with left-sided colitis (69%) or proctitis (60%), (controls 31%). The results of our own study agree with these findings. We found that DR2 was more frequent in the total colitis group (43%) than the distal colitis group (29%) or controls (30%). Indeed, a combined analysis (Woolf-Haldane), of the three previously reported studies of DR antigens in ulcerative colitis [25, 26, 28], plus our own results, confirms a significant association with DR2 ($\chi^2 = 20.7$, $p < 0.001$). However, χ^2 for heterogeneity was also significant ($\chi^2 = 18.0$, $p < 0.001$).

Conclusions

There may be an association between Crohn's disease or ulcerative colitis and various HLA antigens but only in some populations or only with certain subgroups. As we have indicated, there are precedents for both these possibilities in previously reported series involving non-gastrointestinal disorders. Any future studies should take these factors into account when they are reported.

References

1   McConnell, R. B.: Genetics and inflammatory bowel disease; in Rachmilewitz, International Symposium on Inflammatory Bowel Disease, Jerusalem 1981. Developments in gastroenterology, vol. 3, pp. 152–160 (Martinus Nijhoff, The Hague 1982).
2   Farmer, R. G.; Michener, W. M.; Sivak, D. S.: Studies of family history in inflammatory bowel disease; in Peña, 2nd International Workshop on Crohn's disease, Noordwijk/Leiden 1980. Developments in gastroenterology, vol. 1, pp. 213–218 (Martinus Nijhoff, The Hague 1981).
3   Lewkonia, R. M.; McConnell, R. B.: Familial inflammatory bowel disease, Heredity or environment? Gut *17:* 235–245 (1976).

4   Kraft, S. C.; Kirsner, J. B.: The immunology of ulcerative colitis and Crohn's disease: clinical and humoral aspects; in Kirsner, Inflammatory bowel disease, pp. 60–80 (Lea & Febiger, Philadelphia 1975).

5   Watson, D. W.; Shorter, R. G.: The immunology of ulcerative colitis and Crohn's disease – cell-mediated immune responses; in Kirsner, Inflammatory bowel disease, pp. 81–98 (Lea & Febiger, Philadelphia 1975).

6   Lagercrantz R.; Perlmann, P.; Hammerstrom, S.: Immunologic studies in ulcerative colitis. V. Family studies. Gastroenterology 60: 381–389 (1971).

7   Thorsby, E.; Lie, S. O.: Relationship between the HL-A system and susceptibility to disease. Transplant. Proc. 3: 1305–1307 (1971).

8   Gleeson, M. H.; Walker, J. S.; Wentzel, J.; Chapman, J. A.; Harris, R.: Human leucocyte antigens in Crohn's disease and ulcerative colitis. Gut 13: 438–440 (1972).

9   Asquith, P.; Mackintosh,P.; Stokes, P. L.; Holmes, G. K. T.; Cooke, W. T.: Histocompatibility antigens in patients with inflammatory bowel disease. Lancet i: 113–115 (1974).

10 Brewerton, D. A.; Caffrey, M.; Nicholls, A.; Walters, D.; James, D. C. O.: HL-A27 and arthropathies associated with ulcerative colitis and psoriasis. Lancet i: 956–958 (1974).

11 Jacoby, R. K.; Jayson, M. I. V.: HL-A27 in Crohn's disease. Ann. rheum. Dis. 33: 422–424 (1974).

12 Korsmeyer, S.; Strickland, R. G.; Wilson, I. D.; Williams, R. C. J. R.: Serum lymphocytotoxic and lymphocytophilic antibody activity in inflammatory bowel disease. Gastroenterology 45: 413–420 (1963).

13 Lewkonia, R. B.; Woodrow, J. C.; McConnell, R. B.; Price Evans, D. A. P.: HL-A antigens in inflammatory bowel disease. Lancet i: 574–575 (1974).

14 Russell, A. S.; Percy, J. S.; Schlaut, J.; Sartor, V. E.; Goodhart, J. M.; Sherbaniuk, R. W.; Kidd, E. G.: Transplantation antigens in Crohn's disease. Dig. Dis. 20: 359–361 (1975).

15 Bergman, L.; Lindblom, J. B.; Safwenberg, J.; Krause, U.: HL-A frequencies in Crohn's disease and ulcerative colitis. Tissue Antigens 7: 145–150 (1976).

16 Mallas, E. G.; Mackintosh, P.; Asquith, P.; Cooke, W. T.: Histocompatibility antigens in inflammatory bowel disease. Gut 17: 906–910 (1976).

17 Nahir, M.; Gideoni, O.; Eidelman, S.; Barzilai, A.: HLA antigens in ulcerative colitis. Lancet ii: 573 (1976).

18 Tsuchiya, M.; Yoshida, H.; Asakura, H.; Hibi, T.; Ono, A.; Mizuno, Y.; Tsuji, K.: HLA antigens and ulcerative colitis in Japan. Digestion 15: 286–294 (1977).

19 Berg-Loonen, E. M.; Dekker-Saeys, B. J.; Meuwissen, S. G. M.; Nijenhuis, L. E.; Engelfriet, C. P.: Histocompatibility antigens and other genetic markers in ankylosing spondylitis and inflammatory bowel diseases. J. Immunogenet. 4: 167–175 (1977).

20 Woodrow, J. C.; Lewkonia, R. M.; McConnell, R. B.; Berg-Loonen, E. M. V. D.; Meuwissen, S. G. M.; Dekker-Saeys, B. J.; Nijenhuis, L. E.; Mowbray, J. F.; Johnson, N. McI.: HLA antigens in inflammatory bowel disease. Tissue Antigens 11: 147–152 (1978).

21 Hiwatashi, N.; Kikuchi, T.; Masamune, O.; Ouchi, E.; Watanabe, H.; Goto, Y.: HLA antigens in inflammatory bowel disease. Tohoku J. exp. Med. 131: 381–385 (1980).

22 Delpre, G.; Kadish, N.; Gazit, E.; Joshua, H.; Zamir, R.: HLA antigens in ulcerative colitis and Crohn's disease in Israel. Gastroenterology 78: 1452–1457 (1980).

23 Eade, O. E.; Moulton, C.; MacPherson, B. R.; Andre-Ukena, S. St.; Albertini, R. J.; Beeken, S. L.: Discordant HLA haplotype segregation in familial Crohn's disease. Gastroenterology 79: 271–275 (1980).

24 Schwartz, S. W.; Siegelbaum, S. P.; Fazio, T. L.; Hubbell, C.; Henry, J. B.: Regional enteritis: evidence for genetic transmission by HLA typing. Ann. intern. Med. *93:* 424–427 (1980).

25 Peña, A. S.; Biemond, I.; Kuiper, G.; Weterman, I. T.; Leeuwen, A. V.; Schreuder, I.; Rood, J. J. V.: HLA antigen distribution and HLA haplotype segregation in Crohn's disease. Tissue Antigens *16:* 56–61 (1980).

26 Burnham, W. R.; Gelsthorpe, K.; Langman, M. J. S.: HLA-D related antigens in inflammatory bowel disease; in Pena, 2nd International Workshop on Crohn's Disease, Noordwijk/Leiden 1980. Developments in gastroenterology, vol. 1, pp. 192–196 (Martinus Nijhoff, The Hague 1981).

27 Cohen, Z.; McCulloch, P.; Leung, M. K.; Mervart, H.: Histocompatibility antigens in patients with Crohn's disease; in Pena, 2nd International Workshop on Crohn's Disease, Norrdwijk/Leiden 1980. Developments in gastroenterology, vol. 1, pp. 186–191 (Martinus Nijhoff, The Hague, 1981).

28 Smolen, J. S.; Gangl, A.; Polterauer, P.; Menzel, E. J.; Mayr, W. R.: HLA antigens in inflammatory bowel disease. Gastroenterology *84:* 34–38 (1982).

29 Asakura, H.; Tsuchiya, M.; Aiso, S.; Watanabe, M.; Kobayashi, K.; Hibi, T.; Ando, K.; Takata, H.; Sekiguchi, S.: Association of the human lymphocyte DR2 antigen with Japanese ulcerative colitis. Gastroenterology *82:* 413–418 (1982).

30 Lehner, T.; Welsh, K. I.; Batchelor, J. R.: The relationship of HLA-B and DR phenotypes to Behcet's syndrome, recurrent oral ulceration and class of immune complexes. Immunology *47:* 581–581 (1982).

31 Chambers, T. J.; Morson, B. C.: the granuloma in Crohn's disease. Gut *20:* 269–274 (1979).

32 Price, A. B.: Overlap in the spectrum of non-specific inflammatory bowel disease 'colitis indeterminate'. J. clin. Path. *31:* 567–577 (1978).

33 Farid, N. R.; Sampson, L.; Noel, E. P.; Barnard, J. M.; Manderville, R.; Larsen, B.; Marshall, W. H.; Carter, N. D.: A study of human leucocyte D. locus related antigens in Graves' disease. J. clin. Invest. *63:* 108–113 (1979).

34 Grumet, F. C.; Payne, R. D.; Konishi, J.; Mori, T.; Kriss, J. P.: HLA antigens in Japanese patients with Graves' disease. Tissue Antigens *6:* 347–352 (1975).

35 Woolf, B.: On estimating the relation between blood group and disease. Ann. hum. Genet. *19:* 251–253 (1955).

36 Haldane, J. B. S.: The estimation and significance of the logarithm of a ratio of frequencies. Ann. hum. Genet. *20:* 309–311 (1955).

37 Swejgaard, A.; Nielsen, L. S.; Svejgaard, E.; Kissmeyer-Nielsen, F.; Hjortschoj, A.; Zachariae, H.: HL-A in psoriasis vulgaris and in pustular psoriasis population and family studies. Br. J. Derm. *91:* 145–153 (1974).

Dr. A. Ellis, Consultant Gastroenterologist, Gastroenterology Unit,
Broadgreen Hospital, Thomas Drive, Liverpool L14 3LB (UK)

Epidemiology

Front. gastrointest. Res., vol. 11, pp. 42–53 (Karger, Basel 1986)

Epidemiological Data of Chronic Inflammatory Bowel Diseases in the Copenhagen Region

Povl Riis, Vibeke Binder

Medical-Gastroenterological Department, Herlev Hospital, University of Copenhagen, Herlev, Denmark

Background for the Study

The County of Copenhagen, except for a small part on the island of Amager, forms a continuous region, comprising in 1962, 460,143 inhabitants and in 1978, 573,237 inhabitants. This area is the background for our epidemiological studies on chronic inflammatory bowel diseases. The population, which is predominantly urban, nevertheless in respect to its social distribution, is in accordance with the general distribution in Denmark [1] where the total population comprises approximately 5.2 million.

An exact registration of the number of persons grouped by age and sex, living in the area exists for each calender year [1] and these figures are the background for the epidemiological figures obtained. Via the Danish National Person Registry, patients who have left the area of Copenhagen County can be traced to other parts of the country or, possible emigration or death.

The Danish national health care system allows people, free of charge, to visit hospitals, out-patients clinics, practising specialists and general practitioners. This had made it possible to collect a group of patients and to establish clinical follow-up at regular intervals.

Study Population

All the patients who, between 1960 and 1978, fulfilled the diagnostic criteria for either ulcerative colitis or Crohn's disease [2] and were living in the above-mentioned Copenhagen County area, were included in the

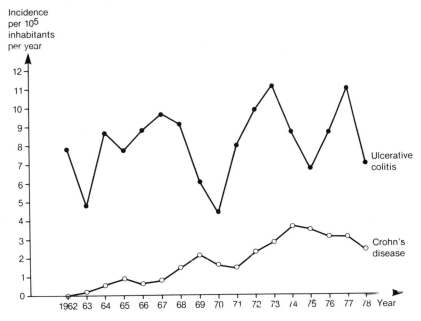

Incidence of ulcerative colitis and Crohn's disease in Copenhagen county 1962–1978

Fig 1. The annual incidence of ulcerative colitis and Crohn's disease in the County of Copenhagen, 1962 to 1978.

study. In all, 783 patients fulfilled the diagnostic criteria for ulcerative colitis and 185 patients for Crohn's disease. By questionnaires to all general practitioners, surgeons, pediatricians and physicians in greater Copenhagen, it was confirmed that our patient group included more than 99% of the patients with a diagnosis of chronic inflammatory bowel diseases in the area [2].

Results

Incidence and Prevalence
The annual *incidence* of ulcerative colitis and Crohn's disease is given in figure 1 and the specific annual incidences in the two sexes separately in figure 2. During the period the annual incidence for women was constant for *ulcerative colitis*, the median being 9.0 per 10^5, while the annual inci-

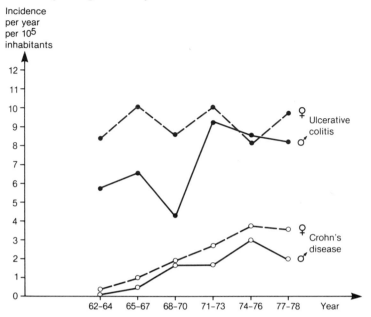

Incidence of ulcerative colitis and Crohn's disease in Copenhagen County 1962-78

Fig. 2. Incidence of ulcerative colitis and Crohn's disease in the County of Copenhagen, 1962 to 1978, in men and women separately. The annual incidences are given as mean of three consecutive years.

dence for men rose from 6.1 to 7.9 per 10^5, from the first to the second half of the study period.

The incidence for *Crohn's disease* rose significantly during the period, being 2.8 per 10^5 inhabitants in the 1970s while only 0.8 per 10^5 in the 1960s. The increase was similar in the two sexes. An apparent plateau from 1974 to 1978 did not reach statistical significance.

The annual incidence of the diseases in different *age groups* is shown in figure 3, given as a mean of the years 1970 to 1978. Incidence peaks were found in ulcerative colitis in age groups 20–35 and 65–70 years, and in Crohn's disease at 20–30 years, while no significant second peak was found here.

The increase in ulcerative colitis incidence in men, in the last half of the study period, is shown in figure 4 to derive from an increase in older age groups especially.

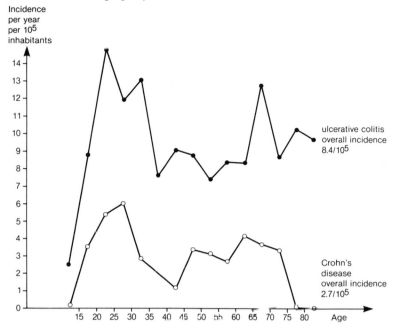

Mean incidence per year (1970–78) per 10^5 inhabitants in different age groups

Fig. 3. Mean annual incidence (1970 to 1978) in different age groups.

The *prevalence* at the end of 1978 was found to be 117 per 10^5 inhabitants for *ulcerative colitis*, 104 for men and 129 for women, comprising both patients from the incidence group who still lived in the area and patients who had moved into the region after their disease had been diagnosed. Operated and non-operated patients were included.

The prevalence for *Crohn's disease* at the end of 1978 was 34 per 10^5 inhabitants, 24 for men and 41 for women.

Clinical Appearance

The *localization* of the disease when diagnosed, is given in figures 5 and 6. Only X-rays and sigmoidoscopy were used for examination and not colonoscopy since it was not available in the first years of the study [3]. In tables I and II the localization of disease is expressed in subgroups, by which the patient group can be divided for further prognostic studies.

The *age* of the patients at time of diagnosis was similar for the two diseases, as shown in table III. The interval from the first symptom to

Table I. Localization of ulcerative colitis at the time of diagnosis

Total colon	16%
Substantial part of colon	43%
Rectum only	41%

Table II. Localization of Crohn's disease at the time of diagnosis

Small bowel only	31%
Large bowel only	28%
Large and small bowel	36%
Duodenal or perianal	5%

Table III. Age of the patients at diagnosis

	Median, years	Range, years
Ulcerative colitis (n = 783)	33.8 F = 34.4; M = 33.0	2–87
Crohn's disease (n = 185)	33.3 F = 33.3; M = 33.3	4–76

Table IV. Length of interval from first symptom to diagnosis

	Median, years	Range, years
Ulcerative colitis (n = 783)	1.7	0–14
Crohn's disease (n = 185)	3.2	0–20

diagnosis, however, was significantly longer in Crohn's disease ($p < 0.05$) (table IV). The length of the interval showed no correlation to the age and sex of the patients, and did not change during the observation period, which could have explained the changes in incidence.

The frequency of different *symptoms* is shown for ulcerative colitis in table V and for Crohn's disease in table VI. The occurrence of symptoms has been analysed in relation to age, sex and localization of disease. There was no correlation between age or sex and symptomatology or

Table V. Symptoms at diagnosis in 783 patients with ulcerative colitis

Bowel habits	
Diarrhoea and bleeding	73%
Diarrhoea without bleeding	5%
Bleeding without diarrhoea	15%
No diarrhoea, no bleeding	7%
Other manifestations	
Abdominal pains and/or rectal cramps	53%
Fever	27%
Weight loss	43%
Immunological manifestations	
Joints and/or skin and/or eyes	13%

Table VI. Symptoms at diagnosis in 185 patients with Crohn's disease

Bowel habits	
Diarrhoea and bleeding	47%
Diarrhoea without bleeding	19%
Bleeding without diarrhoea	4%
No diarrhoea, no bleeding	30%
Other manifestations	
Abdominal pains and/or rectal cramps	76%
Fever	34%
Weight loss	54%
Fistulae/abscesses	23%
Immunological manifestations	
Joints and/or skin and/or eyes	12%

localization of ulcerative colitis. In Crohn's disease the intestinal symptoms were independent of the age and sex of the patients whereas abdominal pains were significantly more frequent in younger age groups (p < 0.01). 84% of the patients less than 45 years old experienced pains, compared to 64% of the patients over that age. There was no correlation between pains and localization of the disease. No other single symptom was related to age or sex of the patients.

The ileal localization of Crohn's disease appeared more often in younger persons (median age 28 years) than sites elsewhere (median age 44 years), but there were no differences between the sexes in that respect. The ileal localization was significantly more often connected to weight loss than were other sites.

Female incidence of ulcerative colitis in different age groups

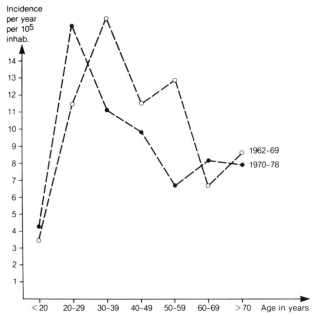

Incidence
per year
per 10^5
inhab.

1962–69
1970–78

< 20   20–29   30–39   40–49   50–59   60–69   > 70   Age in years

Male incidence of ulcerative colitis in different age groups

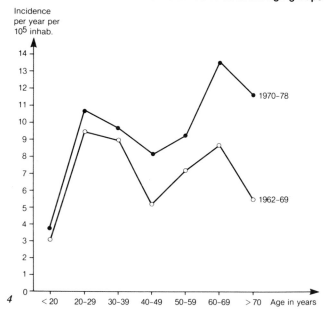

Incidence
per year per
10^5 inhab.

1970–78

1962–69

< 20   20–29   30–39   40–49   50–59   60–69   > 70   Age in years

4

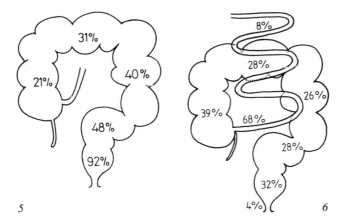

5   6

Fig. 5. Localization of disease at diagnosis, in 783 patients with ulcerative colitis.

Fig. 6. Localization of disease at diagnosis, in 185 patients with Crohn's disease; given as percentage of patients with inflammatory changes in each separate segment of the gastrointestinal tract.

Eventual Course of the Diseases

In the follow-up period where the patients were seen regularly and at least annually, each observation year was considered and characterized according to disease activity, working capacity, operation, medical treatment and length of time admitted to hospital. On the background of these variables *critical events* were defined, and the eventual course was analysed in relation to the clinical appearance of the disease at diagnosis [4, 5].

Influenced by vigorous medical and, or, surgical treatment the *survival* of patients with Crohn's disease and women with ulcerative colitis was similar to that of the background population (fig. 7, 8). Men with ulcerative colitis, appeared to have a slight excess mortality in the year of diagnosis and the following year, but not later in the course [4, 5] (fig. 9).

The principles of *treatment* have been salazosulphapyridine in doses of 2–3 g/day, as a long-term treatment in ulcerative colitis, combined with a series of short intensive steroid treatments of a few months' duration if there was a clinical effect. The starting dose used was 1–2 mg/kg body weight per day. If no effect, the patients underwent colectomy within 1–2 weeks after start of steroid treatment.

Fig. 4. Mean female and male annual incidence in the first and second half of the study period in ten year age periods. No significant difference in age of women in the two periods. Significantly higher incidence for men over 60 years of age in the second half of the study.

Survival Crohn's disease – both sexes

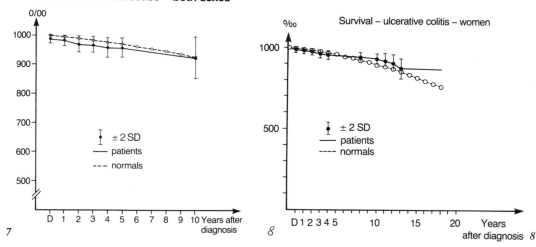

Fig. 7. Survival of patients with Crohn's disease compared with the age- and sex-matched background population.

Fig. 8. Survival of female patients with ulcerative colitis compared with the age-matched female background population ('normals').

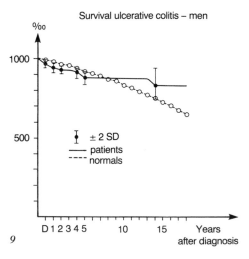

Fig. 9. Survival of male patients with ulcerative colitis compared with the age-matched male background population ('normals').

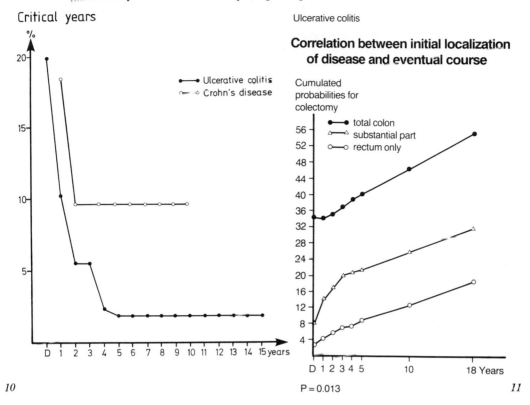

Fig. 10. Occurrence of *critical events* in ulcerative colitis and Crohn's disease in relation to duration of the disease.

Fig. 11. The cumulative probabilities of being colectomized, having total colon, substantial part of colon, or rectum only involved at the time of diagnosis.

Ten percent of the patients with ulcerative colitis were colectomized within the year of diagnosis, 2–3% the following year, and from the 4th year 1% per year were operated. Cumulative colectomy rates after 10, 15, and 18 years with the disease were 23, 28 and 31%, respectively.

In Crohn's disease salazosulphapyridine was given to patients who tolerated the drug, in doses of 2–3 g/day. Steroid treatment has been used in flare-up periods in short treatment courses of a few months' duration, starting with doses of 1 mg/kg body weight and quickly reduced to 10–15 mg/day. In cases with medical failure limited intestinal resections have been carried out. Cumulative operation rates after 10 years with Crohn's disease were 42% operated once, 13% twice or more; 45% of the patients were not operated on at all.

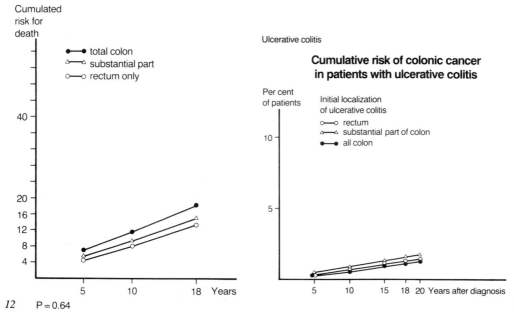

P = 0.64

Fig. 12. Cumulative risks of death, having total colon, substantial part of colon, or rectum only involved at the time of diagnosis.

Fig. 13. Cumulative risk of developing large bowel cancer, having total colon, substantial part of colon, or rectum only involved at the time of diagnosis.

In ulcerative colitis the frequency of *critical events* diminished rapidly during the first few years, while in Crohn's disease the risk seems to be constant, about 10% per year from the second year after the diagnosis (fig. 10).

In *ulcerative colitis* the only primary factor with influence on the long-term prognosis was extent of disease which was found to influence the possibility of colectomy significantly, but not the probability of death or occurrence of cancer (fig. 11–13).

In *Crohn's disease* there was no significant difference between the eventual outcome of the disease, whether it was localized in small bowel, large bowel or both, at diagnosis. Generally male patients run a more critical course than female, and patients who had continuous symptoms, in the year of diagnosis and the first year thereafter, showed a more severe long-term course than patients with an intermittent course during that period.

The cumulative risk of developing *cancer* in the large bowel in *ulcerative colitis* was found to be 1.4% (95% significance limits 0.7–2.8%) after 18 years with the disease. The risk of large bowel cancer was of the same magnitude whether the patient had total colon, substantial part of the colon or only rectum involved at the time of diagnosis (fig. 13). Patients with total colon involvement primarily, were colectomized more often than patients with only substantial or rectal involvement, thus diminishing the number of patients at risk in that group. The cumulative risk of gastrointestinal cancer in *Crohn's disease*, after 10 years, was estimated to be 0.6% (95% confidence limits 0.10–3.1%).

References

1   Danmarks Statistik (Denmark's Central Statistical Agency): Annual tables, Copenhagen: 1962–1968

2   Binder, V.; Both, H.; Hansen, P. K.; Hendriksen, C.; Kreiner, S.; Torp-Pedersen, K.: Incidence and prevalence of ulcerative colitis and Crohn's disease in the County of Copenhagen, 1962 to 1978. Gastroenterology *83:* 563–568 (1982).

3   Both, H.; Torp-Pedersen, K.; Kreiner, S.; Hendriksen, C.; Binder, V.: Clinical appearance at diagnosis of ulcerative colitis and Crohn's disease in a regional patient group. Scand. J. Gastroent. *18:* 987–991 (1983).

4   Hendriksen, C.; Kreiner, S.; Binder, V.: The long-term prognosis in ulcerative colitis – based on results from a regional patient group from the County of Copenhagen. Gut *26:* 158–163 (1985).

5   Binder, V.; Hendriksen, C.; Kreiner, S.: The prognosis in Crohn's disease based on results from a regional patient group from the County of Copenhagen. Gut *26:* 146–150 (1985).

Vibeke Binder, MD, Medical-Gastroenterological Department C,
Herlev University Hospital, DK-2730 Herlev (Denmark)

Front. gastrointest. Res., vol. 11, pp. 54–57 (Karger, Basel 1986)

Epidemiology of Inflammatory Bowel Disease in The Netherlands

S. Shivananda, I. T. Weterman, A. S. Peña

Department of Gastroenterology,
University Hospital, Leiden, The Netherlands

Introduction

There has been no systematic epidemiological study of inflammatory bowel disease (IBD) in The Netherlands; hence there is no reliable data on its incidence and prevalence or about the host and environmental risk factors operating in the country that make the Dutch population susceptible to this disease. Part of the problem is that there is no uniform system of medical information for in-patient and out-patient services which can be readily used for epidemiological investigations. This is despite the fact that the Dutch health care system is one of the most comprehensive and egalitarian systems in Western Europe and stands out well in many parameters of effectiveness, and the process as well as the outcome of medical care [1–3].

To overcome this dearth in knowledge, the authors are presently engaged in an epidemiological investigation of IBD in the Leiden health care region of the Netherlands. Until firm data becomes available through this study, the investigators have used the following sources:

(1) Hospital discharge data produced by the 'Stichting Medische Registratie' (SMR) Utrecht. This is a national organization of hospital utilization statistics similar to the hospital discharge reporting system in the United States known as the Professional Activity Study (PAS). The SMR maintains a bank of information on discharges for nearly 95% of the hospitals in the country using the International Classification of Disease code (ICD) as proposed by the World Health Organization (WHO).

(2) Results of a sample survey of IBD case-load carried by medical specialists on their in- and out-patients roster.

Table I. Prevalence of ulcerative colitis and Crohn's disease according to The Netherlands hospital discharge rate 1977–1981[1]

Year	Estimated[2] Population per 10^6	Ulcerative colitis		Crohn's disease	
		total number	per 10^5	total number	per 10^5
1977	13.9	856	6.2	1,203	8.7
1978	14.0	876	6.3	1,320	9.4
1979	14.0	846	6.0	1,346	9.6
1980	14.1	1,040	7.4	1,398	9.9
1981	14.2	977	6.9	1,384	9.7

[1] Source: Stichting Medische Registratie, Utrecht.
[2] Estimated population source: Central Bureau of Statistics (CBS) Statistisch Zakboek 1977–1981, Staatsuitgeverij, Den Haag.

Hospital Discharge Data

The hospital discharge data is of limited utility in assessing the incidence and prevalence of disease in a population. Ordinarily it represents: (a) the hospital admission rate in a disease category; (b) a partial measure of cases with disease severity which must be hospitalized for treatment, and (c) physician behaviour or financial incentives to hospitalize. Then, of course, there is the problem that not all the hospitals in the country may be members of a hospital information system; problem of multiple admissions of the patient for the same condition; and most importantly who is doing the ICD coding: the physician in-charge of case management or the clerk in the medical registration department of a hospital. Despite these limitations, the hospital discharge data has proven to be a very useful tool in epidemiological studies [4–6]. In fact, in some situations this may be the only data available for estimating disease frequency in a population. The data shown in table I provides estimates of IBD frequency in the Dutch population over a 5-year period between 1977 and 1981 based on hospital discharge data. Further analysis of these data along with age and sex distribution, shows that the risk of developing IBD in The Netherlands is greatest in the third decade of life for both sexes, as suggested by *Kyle and Stark* [7] in their 1971 investigation for Scotland, and then there appears to be a slight preponderance of females in the IBD population.

Table II. Province of Zuid-Holland: IBD case-load, 1982, based on a 42% reponse rate of relevant specialists

	Crohn's disease cases		Ulcerative colitis cases		Total IBD
	all	new	all	new	
Internists, paediatricians, and gastroenterologists (n = 112)	1,008	121	569	112	1,577
Prevalence per 10^5	32.3	3.8	18.2	3.6	50.5

Sample Survey of Specialist Medical Practices

A sample survey of 265 hospital specialists working in the field of IBD (internists and paediatricians) was carried out by the authors in the province of Zuid-Holland. A simple mail questionnaire combined with random personal interviews to check the validity and reliability of information was used. Specialists were asked to provide an estimate of the case-load they were carrying in their in- and out-patients roster under the diagnostic label of Crohn's disease (CD) and ulcerative colitis (UC) in 1982. The survey was carried out in early 1983. From the 265 contacted 112 responded, i.e. a response rate of 42%. The results are shown in table II.

With an estimated population of 3,121,500 in 1982 in the Province of Zuid-Holland these numbers suggested a period prevalence of 32.3 and an incidence of 4 cases of CD per 100,000 population. If this can be confirmed by a systematic epidemiological study now under way, this will put The Netherlands closer to the Welsh [4] and Stockholm [8] experience. For UC, these data suggest a period prevalence of 18, and an incidence rate of 3.6 cases per 10^5. The authors realize that these data are inconclusive at present.

Conclusions

At the moment there are no firm epidemiological data on IBD in The Netherlands. The hospital discharge data of SMR covering a 5-year period between 1977 and 1981 and a sample survey of medical specialists carried out by the authors provides some indication of IBD epidemiology in The Netherlands. These data should be regarded as working estimates of IBD frequency; not much more. The epidemiological study now in progress will throw more definitive light on the situation in The Netherlands.

References

1 Cochrane, A. L.: Effectiveness and efficiency; in Cochrane, Random reflections on health services, pp. 15–65 (Nuffield Provincial Hospitals Trust, London 1972).
2 Williamson, J. W.: Assessing and improving health care outcomes; in Balinger, The health accounting approach to quality assurance, pp. 25–68 (Cambridge, 1978).
3 Donabedian, A.: Promoting quality through evaluating the process of patient care. Med. Care 6: 181–202 (1968).
4 Mayberry, J. F.; Rhodes, J.; Newcombe, R. G.: Crohn's disease in Wales, 1967–1977. An epidemiological survey based on hospital admissions. Post-grad. med. J. 56: 336–341 (1980).
5 Monk, M.; Mendelhoff, A. I.; Siegel, C. J.; Lilienfield, A.: An epidemiological study of ulcerative colitis and regional enteritis among adults in Baltimore. Gastroenterology 53: 198–200 (1967).
6 Garland, C. F.; Lilienfeld, A. M.; Mendelhoff, I. A.; Markowitz, J. A.; Terrell, K. B.; Garland, F. C.: Incidence rates of ulcerative colitis and Crohn's disease in fifteen areas of the United States. Gastroenterology 83: 1115–1124 (1981).
7 Kyle, J., Stark, J.: Fall in the incidence of CD. Gut 21: 340–343 (1980).
8 Hellers, G.: Some epidemiological aspects of CD in Stockholm Country 1955–1979; in Peña, Weterman, Strober, Booth, Recent advances in Crohn's disease, pp. 158–162 (Martinus Nijhoff, The Hague 1981).

S. Shivananda, MD, Department of Gastroenterology, University Hospital, Rijnsburgweg 10, NL-2333 AA Leiden (The Netherlands)

Front. gastrointest. Res., vol. 11, pp. 58–67 (Karger, Basel 1986)

Local Variations of Prevalence of Crohn's Disease in the Mersey Region

Bryan F. Warren, Richard B. McConnell

Gastroenterology Unit, Broadgreen Hospital, Liverpool, UK

The prevalence of inflammatory bowel disease in western countries is thought to be patchy, but no pattern has been detected. In some areas there is an impression that whilst the incidence of Crohn's disease is still rising, that of ulcerative colitis has not been doing so to the same extent [1–6]. In Aberdeen and Stockholm County there is evidence that Crohn's disease may have reached a plateau of incidence [7, 8].

We have conducted two studies of patients in the Mersey region. The first is an analysis of a computer file of 246 patients with inflammatory bowel disease, who during the years 1967–1980 attended the Gastroenterology Unit of Broadgreen Hospital, one of the Gastroenterology Units in Liverpool. This series is quite separate from the patients reported by *Lewkonia and McConnell* [9] from the Liverpool Royal Infirmary. The second is a geographical analysis of Hospital Activity Analysis (HAA) data of the Mersey Region for the period 1974–1980 for Crohn's disease. In this study, comparison is made with coeliac patients' data for the same period.

Analysis of Broadgreen Hospital Patients

The Broadgreen Hospital Gastroenterology Unit computer file was the whole source of information used in this analysis of 109 cases of Crohn's disease and 137 cases of ulcerative colitis who had been referred to the Unit between 31st October, 1967 and 4th February, 1980. The general pattern of referral of cases to the Unit is one of increase and during most years there were more new cases of ulcerative colitis than Crohn's disease. Only from 1974 to 1976 were there more Crohn's cases than colitis (fig. 1).

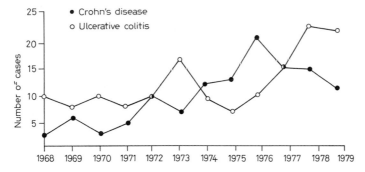

Fig. 1. Graph showing the number of new cases seen each year (1968–1979).

Table I. Age at first consultation

Age group, years	Crohn's disease		Ulcerative colitis	
	n	%	n	%
10–19	19	17.4	14	10.2
20–29	27	24.8	20	14.6
30–39	28	25.6	34	24.8
40–49	13	11.9	20	14.6
50–59	9	8.3	22	16.1
60–69	9	8.3	16	11.7
Over 70	4	3.7	11	8.0

Age at First Consultation

From the data available it was not possible to establish the precise age of onset, but age at first consultation is probably fairly closely related (table I). The majority of the patients with Crohn's disease presented slightly earlier in life than the majority of those with ulcerative colitis. There is little difference between the age of presentation of males and females with either disease. The mean age of presentation of patients with Crohn's disease was 32.6 years for males and 37.2 years for females. For ulcerative colitis it was 41.2 years for males and 42.4 years for females. We could not demonstrate in these data any second peak of onset in Crohn's disease which has been reported by some [10, 11] although this has been suggested by *Hellers* [12] to probably be an artefact caused by too few cases in the higher age group.

Table II. IBD patients of various social classes

Social class	Crohn's disease		Weighted control		Ulcerative colitis		Weighted control	
	n	%	n	%	n	%	n	%
I	6	6.4	385	5.2	8	9.3	195	5.1
II	19	20.4	1,228	16.5	17	19.8	598	15.6
III N	20	21.5	1,770	23.7	18	20.9	1,013	26.4
III M	30	32.3	1,999	26.8	27	31.4	955	24.9
IV	13	14.0	1,368	18.3	10	11.6	721	18.8
V	5	5.4	709	9.5	6	7.0	352	9.2
Total	93	100.0	7,459	100.0	86	100.0	3,834	100.0

Sex Distribution

No significant overall sex difference was found, the percentage of females being 57.8% in our Crohn's group and 53.2% in the ulcerative colitis group. Differences in sex distribution of cases of Crohn's disease have varied from survey to survey, but overall are roughly equal [13, 14].

Social Class

The occupations of the patients had been classified according to the Registrar General's classification of occupations [15]. A control has been calculated for both diseases, weighted according to the number of patients with that disease in each postcode area. The social class distribution of each postcode area was calculated from the proportion contributed to each by its constituent electoral wards, when the boundaries of both electoral wards and postcode areas were plotted on the same map. Social class structure of the electoral wards came from the 1971 Census data [16–18]. Where a postcode area contributed only 1 patient with a particular disease, it was ignored when calculating the weighted control and the patient was omitted from the calculations. Also excluded were patients whose homes were outside the Mersey Hospital Region. This led to 16 patients out of 109 with Crohn's disease being excluded from this part of the study and 51 out of 137 patients with ulcerative colitis. The social class distribution of the patients and their weighted controls are given in table II. There is no significant difference between the social class distribution of the group of patients with Crohn's disease and its weighted control, nor between the ulcerative colitis group and its control. This is in keeping with most other studies [19], though some studies have indicated the patients to have higher education achievements than their controls [11, 20, 21].

Table III. IBD referrals, as percentages of referrals of all gastrointestinal disorders to the Unit from postal districts which have referred more than 50 patients during this period of study (1967–1980)

Postcode area	Total number referred	Crohn's disease		Ulcerative colitis	
		n	%	n	%
L4	300	–	–	3	1.00
L5	211	1	0.47	–	–
L6	466	4	0.86	12	2.58
L7	265	2	0.75	6	2.25
L9	77	2	2.60	–	–
L10	57	–	–	1	1.75
L11	373	2	0.54	7	1.88
L12	556	1	0.19	8	1.44
L13	962	4	0.42	7	0.73
L14	906	9	0.99	10	1.10
L15	314	5	1.59	3	0.96
L16	334	5	1.49	6	1.80
L17	129	2	1.59	–	–
L18	189	3	1.59	–	–
L19	158	1	0.63	3	1.89
L21	64	–	–	2	3.13
L23	91	4	4.40	1	1.10
L24	139	4	2.88	3	2.16
L25	774	5	0.65	12	1.55
L27	231	1	0.43	6	2.58
L28	275	3	1.09	1	0.36
L36	596	3	0.50	9	1.50
St. Helens	111	2	1.80	1	0.90
Southport	155	4	2.58	4	2.58
Wirral	178	5	2.81	7	3.93
Runcorn	98	5	5.10	5	5.10
N. E. Wales	173	7	4.04	2	1.16

Geographical Distribution

The percentages of patients with Crohn's disease and ulcerative colitis of the total referrals from each postcode area, during the period 1967–1980, are given in table III. The postcode areas adjoining Broadgreen Hospital (L14, 15, 16, 17, 18) show similar percentages of referrals from Crohn's disease. However, the district with the highest percentage of Crohn's disease, amongst the patients referred to the Broadgreen Unit, was Runcorn. Merseyside postcode areas with a higher relative prevalence of Crohn's disease than ulcerative colitis, those in which the relative prevalences are equal and those in which the relative prevalence of ulcerative colitis is higher are indicated in figure 2.

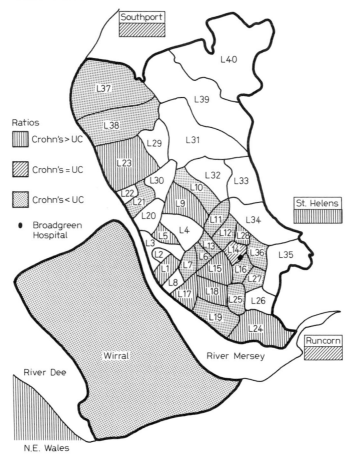

Fig. 2. Map of Merseyside postal districts showing the relative prevalence of Crohn's disease and ulcerative colitis patients attending Broadgreen Hospital.

In general, more patients with ulcerative colitis than Crohn's disease (93 ulcerative colitis to 53 Crohn's) were referred from Liverpool, whereas more cases of Crohn's disease than ulcerative colitis were referred from the peripheral postcode areas. This is almost certainly due to selection, with the disease which is more difficult clinically being referred longer distances, rather than representing a higher proportion of Crohn's disease than ulcerative colitis in rural areas. Even so, the possible high

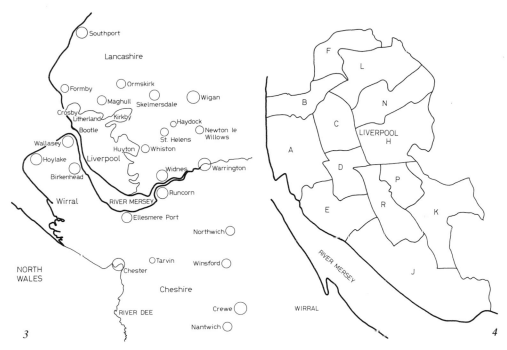

Fig. 3. Map of Mersey Health Region showing location of towns around Liverpool.
Fig. 4. Map showing Liverpool Social Service Districts.

prevalence of both Crohn's disease and ulcerative colitis in Runcorn seems to deserve further investigation, especially because most patients from this Cheshire town, 15 miles from Liverpool (fig. 3), have been re-ferred to hospitals in the centre of Liverpool rather than to Broadgreen Hospital.

Hospital Activity Analysis Data

Hospital Activity Analysis (HAA) data are confined to in-patients. The patients are coded according to the Social Services District in which their home is situated. Population estimates for 1978, in standard age groups, are available for each of these districts, varying from about 50,000 in towns or cities to 10,000 or less in some rural districts. It was thought that the diagnosis of Crohn's disease in HAA data is likely to be

Table IV. Number of hospital discharges, 1974–1980, per 100,000 population of Social Service Districts

District	Population × 1,000	Crohn's disease		Coeliac disease	
		No. per 100,000		No. per 100,000	
		n		n	
Liverpool					
A	37.3	15	40	17	46
B	29.4	19	65	8	27
C	55.6	35	63	17	31
D	47.4	21	44	20	42
E	49.5	30	61	14	28
F	27.9	24	86	6	22
H	64.7	32	49	12	19
J	50.6	25	49	13	26
K	51.7	25	48	15	29
L	39.8	35	88	8	20
N	28.3	10	35	9	32
P	15.0	14	93	3	20
R	30.8	28	91	4	13
Merseyside North of Mersey					
Huyton	61.1	17	28	25	41
Kirkby U. D.	56.7	34	60	37	65
St. Helens C. B.	103.9	42	40	15	14
Haydock U. D.	15.8	4	25	5	32
Newton-le-Willows	21.0	10	48	3	14
Bootle	64.0	24	38	15	23
Southport	88.0	40	45	7	8
Crosby M. B.	56.9	27	47	11	19
Formby U. D.	25.6	11	43	4	16
West Lancs R. D.	44.4	23	52	3	7
Litherland U. D.	22.4	12	54	7	31
Whiston R. D.	84.2	24	28	24	28

accurate and there is no reason to suppose that any degree of error would be more marked in one district than another. Over a 6-year period, the proportion of Crohn's patients who are admitted should be high and similar in all districts. It was therefore decided to study the 1974–1980 HAA data of the Mersey Regional Health Authority for Crohn's disease. As a reference disease it was decided to use coeliac disease which has a higher prevalence in the population, though a lower admission threshold, and which can be expected to have a uniform prevalence throughout the region, expect perhaps in those towns with a large proportion of people of Irish extraction.

Table IV. (Cont.)

District	Population × 1,000	Crohn's disease No. per 100,000		Coeliac disease No. per 100,000	
Merseyside South of Mersey		n		n	
Birkenhead	133.4	65	49	27	20
Wallasey	94.0	75	80	13	14
Bebington	60.0	29	48	10	17
Hoylake	30.9	15	49	0	0
Wirral U. D.	18.7	5	27	5	27
Ellesmere Port	66.1	35	53	19	29
Cheshire					
Chester C. B.	58.4	35	60	11	19
Chester R. D.	38.0	22	58	7	18
Tarvin R. D.	19.4	7	36	5	26
Crewe M. B.	47.1	25	53	1	2
Nantwich R. D.	37.6	16	43	2	5
Winsford U. D.	26.5	11	42	6	23
Northwich R. D.	46.5	22	47	4	9
Runcorn U. D.	61.2	25	41	17	28
Runcorn R. D.	34.9	22	63	10	29
Widnes M. B.	53.6	28	52	10	19
Warrington C. B.	57.5	22	38	8	14

It was possible to identify patients admitted to hospital more than once, even if they had been admitted to different hospitals, by their date of birth and record number. Therefore, the number of individuals with the two diseases, discharged from Mersey Regional Health Authority hospitals during the 6-years period, was found. From the eastern half of Cheshire, patients may have been admitted to Manchester Hospitals, but otherwise few patients living in the region would have been admitted to non-Mersey Regional Health Authority Hospitals. In table IV is given the number of patients per 100,000 population in social service districts at the time of the study omitting those of Eastern Cheshire and those with a population of less than 15,000. With one or two exceptions, the prevalence of Crohn's disease is similar from area to area. The exceptions, however, are rather surprising. Birkenhead and Wallasey on the Wirral (fig. 3) have a similar socio-economic structure and both are fairly industrial areas, yet Crohn's disease appears to be relatively more prevalent in Wallasey than in Birkenhead at the time of our study. We cannot, as yet, offer any reasonable explanation of this. Also two adjacent Social Service

Districts (fig. 4) in the north-east of Liverpool (F & L) and two in the south of Liverpool (P & R) appear to have a higher relative prevalence of Crohn's disease than the other Liverpool districts.

In this study, ascertainment is incomplete for Crohn's disease and more so for coeliac disease, since patients who were diagnosed prior to 1974 and had not been admitted by 1980 will not have been included. It cannot be assumed from the figures, therefore, that Crohn's disease is more prevalent than coeliac disease, since Crohn's patients are more likely to undergo admission than coeliacs who, if they are diagnosed prior to 1974, are unlikely to have been admitted during the period of our study. These data, however, give an indication of relative prevalence of the two diseases in the different areas. From these data there appears to be a tendency for urban districts to have a higher prevalence of Crohn's disease than rural districts, which has been described in some earlier studies [10], but not in others [22]. Runcorn rural district shows a fairly high relative prevalence of Crohn's disease in this study also, but, oddly, the urban district shows a slightly lower relative prevalence. There is only one area which shows a disproportionately high relative prevalence of coeliac disease, which is the urban district of Kirkby to the north of Liverpool. Apart from this the relative prevalence of coeliac disease varies, as one might expect, in a random fashion.

Conclusion

These data from two separate sources, seem to indicate that geographical clustering of patients with Crohn's disease is worthy of further study in the Mersey Region, although clustering was not demonstrated after detailed study elsewhere [23].

References

1   Miller, D.; Keighley, A.; Langman, M.: Changing patterns in the epidemiology of Crohn's disease. Lancet *ii:* 691–693 (1974).
2   Mayberry, J.; Rhodes, J.; Hughes, L.: Incidence of Crohn's disease in Cardiff between 1934 and 1977. Gut *20:* 602–608 (1979).
3   Gilat, T.; Rozen, P.: Epidemiology of Crohn's disease, trends and clues; in Peña, Weterman, Booth, Strober, Recent advances in Crohn's disease (Martinus Nijhoff, The Hague 1981).
4   Brahme, F.; Linström, C.; Wenckert, A.: Crohn's disease in a defined population. Scand. J. Gastroent. *69:* 342–354 (1975).
5   Bergman, L.; Krause, U.: The incidence of Crohn's disease in central Sweden. Scand. J. Gastroent. *10:* 725–729 (1975).

6 Smith, L.; Young, S.; Gillespie, G.; O'Connor, J.; Bell, J.: Epidemiological aspects of Crohn's disease in Clydesdale 1961–1970. Gut *16:* 62–67 (1975).

7 Kyle, J.; Starke, G.: Fall in the incidence of Crohn's disease. Gut *21:* 340–343 (1980).

8 Hellers, G.: Epidemiology of Crohn's disease in Stockholm County; in Pena, Weterman, Booth, Strober, Recent advances in Crohn's disease (Martinus Nijhoff, The Hague 1981).

9 Lewkonia, R.; McConnell, R. B.: Familial inflammatory bowel disease – heredity of or environment? Gut *17:* 235–243 (1976).

10 Kyle, J.: An epidemiological study of Crohn's disease in North East Scotland. Gastroenterology *61:* 826–833 (1971).

11 Rogers, B.; Clark, L.; Virone, J.: The epidemiological and demographic characteristics of inflammatory bowel disease. An analysis of a computerised file of 1,400 patients. J. chron. Dis. *24:* 743–773 (1971).

12 Hellers, G.: Crohn's disease in Stockholm County; in Lee, Crohn's Workshop, p. 90 (H & M Publishers, London 1981).

13 Mendeloff, A.: Epidemiology and socioeconomic factors; in Kirsner, Shorter, Inflammatory bowel disease, p. 13 (Lea & Febiger, Philadelphia 1980).

14 Langman, M.; Burnham, W.: Epidemiology of inflammatory bowel disease; in Allan, Keighley, Alexander-Williams, Hawkins, Inflammatory bowel disease, p. 20 (Churchill-Livingstone, Edinburgh 1983).

15 Classification of Occupations (HMSO, London 1970).

16 Census 1971: England and Wales, Economic activity sub-regional tables (10% sample), tab. 4, pp. 279–282 (HMSO, London 1976).

17 Census 1971: England and Wales, Economic Activity County leaflet, Cheshire (HMSO, London 1975).

18 Census 1971. England and Wales, Economic Activity County leaflet, Lancashire (HMSO, London 1975).

19 Langman, M.: Chronic non-specific inflammatory bowel disease; in Langman, Epidemiology of chronic digestive diseases, p. 85 (Edward Arnold, London 1979).

20 Monk, M.; Mendeloff, A.; Siegel, C.; Lilienfeld, A.: An epidemiological study of ulcerative colitis and regional enteritis among adults in Baltimore. Gastroenterology *56:* 843–857 (1969).

21 Bonnevie, O.: A socioeconomic study of patients with ulcerative colitis Scand. J. Gastroent. *2:* 129–136 (1967).

22 Hellers, G.: Crohn's disease in Stockholm County, 1955–1974. A study of epidemiology, results of surgical treatment and long-term prognosis. Acta chir. Scand., suppl. 490, pp. 1–84 (1979).

23 Miller, D.; Keighley, A.; Smith, P.; Hughes, A.; Langman, M.: Crohn's disease in Nottingham. A search for time-space clustering. Gut *16:* 454–457 (1975)

Dr. R. B. McConnell, 2 Countisbury Drive, Liverpool L16 OJJ (UK)

Front. gastrointest. Res., vol. 11, pp. 68–72 (Karger, Basel 1986)

Prevalence of Chronic Inflammatory Bowel Disease in British Children

Anne Ferguson, Edith A Rifkind, Caroline M Doig

Gastro-Intestinal Unit, Western General Hospital, Edinburgh, UK; Department of Paediatric Surgery, Booth Hall Children's Hospital, Manchester, UK

Introduction

Chronic inflammatory bowel disease in a child or adolescent presents a number of clinical problems additional to those which occur in adults with these diseases. There may be considerable delay in diagnosis; growth failure and retarded sexual development are common; Crohn's disease in young people tends to follow a more aggressive course, as assessed by the rate of post-operative recurrence and mortality; and the malignant potential of ulcerative colitis is higher when there is onset in childhood [1, 2]. This information has been derived from reports of children and adolescents attending paediatric gastroenterology clinics in specialist teaching hospitals such as the Mayo Clinic, Mount Sinai and St. Bartholomew's. There are no good accounts of the patterns of inflammatory bowel disease in general paediatric practice and, indeed, the prevalence of these incurable diseases in children is unknown. We have therefore carried out a study, on behalf of the British Paediatric Gastroenterology Group, in an attempt to establish the prevalence of Crohn's disease and of idiopathic ulcerative colitis, in children in Britain.

Methods

Information on Patients

A letter, explaining the objectives of this study, was sent to all members of the British Paediatric Association, the British Society for Gastroenterology and the British Association of Paediatric Surgeons. Information was sought on patients with inflammatory bowel disease who had been born since January 1964. We requested the name, sex, hospital, hospital

Table I. Patients reported to the childhood IBD investigation

Diagnosis	Male	Female	Total
Crohn's disease	261	186	447
Ulcerative colitis	157	148	305
Not stated, unclassified, other colitides			
	19	15	34

number, year of birth, year of diagnosis and the consultant's working diagnosis (Crohn's disease, idiopathic ulcerative colitis, indeterminate inflammatory bowel disease or other diagnosis). In some instances consultants expressed concern about confidentiality, in which case either the date of birth and sex, or the first three letters of the surname were provided. In order to avoid duplicate registration of the same patient, the results were assembled alphabetically and then filed by the consultant's Regional Health Authority or country

Population Statistics

The office of Populations, Censuses and Surveys provided estimates of the populations of Scotland, Northern Ireland, Wales and the Health Authority regions of England, in the age groups concerned.

Scottish Hospitals In-Patient Statistics

This type of survey will detect only a proportion of the overall number of cases of the diseases under study. We have estimated the magnitude of this error by using Scottish Hospital in-patients data. In Scotland, the Common Services Agency collects information on all in-patients, including diagnosis. Linkage of records takes account of multiple admissions of the same patient. A printout was provided to us, covering the years 1967–1979, and listing patients in whom a diagnosis of either Crohn's disease or ulcerative colitis had been made. The first admission to a hospital in Scotland was taken as date of diagnosis, and only patients born since 1st January 1964 were included in our analysis. The patient's name was omitted from the printout and the consultant concerned was identified only by a numerical code.

Results

A total of 219 forms were returned, many of which contained information from a group rather than from a single gastroenterologist or paediatrician. A total of 447 patients with Crohn's disease and 305 with ulcerative colitis were reported (table I). In the majority of these children the diagnosis had been made between the ages of 8 and 16 years (fig. 1). There were equal numbers of boys and girls with ulcerative colitis, but an excess of males reported to have Crohn's disease. A bias towards the reporting of recently diagnosed patients was obvious (fig. 2); that this was simply bias is shown by the Scottish data which did not reveal any striking

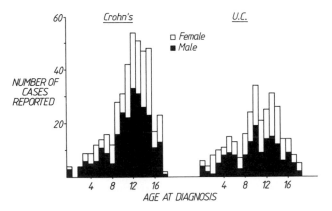

Fig. 1. Age at diagnosis of children reported to the IBD Investigation.

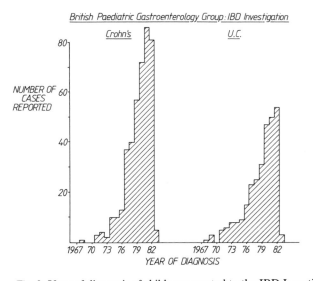

Fig. 2. Year of diagnosis of children reported to the IBD Investigation.

change in incidence of Crohn's disease, and possibly a fall in the incidence of ulcerative colitis (fig. 3).

A breakdown of cases from Scotland, Wales, Northern Ireland and the regions of England is given in table II. As can be seen, there was wide variation in the reported prevalence with high figures for the North Western region, and North East Thames. This is accounted for by high returns from specialist paediatric gastroenterology units.

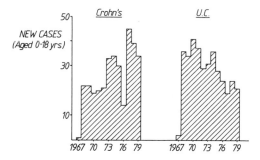

Fig. 3. Numbers of children (new cases) with Crohn's disease or ulcerative colitis, admitted to hospitals in Scotland between 1968 and 1979.

Table II. Distribution, within the UK, of reported patients

Country or RHA	Crohn's disease	Ulcerative colitis	Population aged 0–18 (thousands)	Prevalence of reported IBD per 100,000 children
Scotland	33	38	1,455.9	4.87
Wales	10	11	759.1	2.77
N. Ireland	3	0	533.4	0.56
North Western	64	34	1,107.3	9.21
Mersey	13	1	691.1	2.02
West Midlands	37	23	1,456.4	4.12
South Western	13	7	794.9	2.52
Oxford	13	14	671.0	4.02
Wessex	23	24	726.8	6.47
East Anglia	13	6	508.6	3.74
Trent	28	25	1,256.9	4.22
Yorkshire	25	21	992.3	4.64
Northern	10	6	847.6	1.89
S. W. Thames	11	10	742.2 ⎤	
S. E. Thames	25	30	920.8 ⎟	7.32
N. E. Thames	100	34	965.7 ⎟	
N. W. Thames	26	21	884.3 ⎦	
Total	447	305	15,314.3	4.91
			(Crohn's disease, 2.92)	
			(ulcerative colitis, 1.99)	

We appreciated that only a proportion of inflammatory bowel disease patients would be identified in this exercise. We, therefore, compared the number of reported cases for Scotland, diagnosed between 1967 and 1979 (33) with the number of cases identified by the analysis of Scottish Hospitals in-patients statistics (114), i.e. 29% report rate. If this is representative of the United Kingdom as a whole, then the true prevalence of Crohn's disease will be 10.07 per 100,000 children, and of ulcerative colitis, 6.86.

Discussion

This investigation was conducted in order to establish the prevalence of chronic inflammatory bowel disease in children in the United Kingdom. We requested very limited information, and used the in-patient data for Scotland as a method of checking the accuracy of the results obtained. We have also accepted the consultant's diagnosis of Crohn's disease, ulcerative colitis or indeterminate colitis. The 752 children with chronic inflammatory bowel disease reported to us probably comprise some 30% of the true number of British children with these disabling, incurable diseases. The prevalence is, therefore, of the same order of magnitude as that for phenylketonuria, beta-thalassaemia, Duchenne's muscular dystrophy or haemophilia A[3].

Acknowledgements

This work was supported by a grant from the Edinburgh Gastrointestinal Trust. We are grateful to Mr. *Keith Flanigan* of the Office of Population Censuses and Surveys, and Dr. *Jennifer Webb* of the Common Services Agency, Edinburgh; and to the many doctors who provided details of patients.

References

1   Ferguson, A.: Chronic diarrhoeal disease in older children; in Hull, Recent advances in paediatrics, pp. 97–136 (Churchill-Livingstone, London 1981).
2   Booth, I. W.; Harries, J. T.: Inflammatory bowel disease in childhood. Gut. *25:* 188–202 (1984).
3   Weatherall, D. J.: The new genetics and clinical medicine (Nuffield Provincial Hospital Trust, London 1982).

Dr. Anne Ferguson, Gastro-Intestinal Unit, Western General Hospital, Edinburgh EH4 2XU (UK)

Front. gastrointest. Res., vol. 11, pp. 73–87 (Karger, Basel 1986)

Changes in the Epidemiology, Clinical Presentation and Behaviour of Inflammatory Bowel Disease Occurring in South-East Scotland

J. H. Entrican, W. Sircus

Gastro-intestinal Unit, University of Edinburgh, Western General Hospital, Edinburgh, UK

Introduction

Medical history has been characterised by the rise and fall of disease processes, often largely uninfluenced by therapeutic intervention. The rising tide of interest in inflammatory bowel disease has resulted in a large accummulation of data on the epidemiological and clinical pattern of these diseases. Because of this and the fact that both idiopathic ulcerative colitis and Crohn's disease have been definitely described only within the last century, makes them particularly suitable for a study of the changing pattern of disease with time.

Changes in the natural history of a disease may occur in its incidence and prevalence, its severity, complications, outcome or response to treatment. However, several factors must be taken into account before ascribing changes in its natural history to those of the disease itself, such as the referral pattern of cases, changes in awareness or specialist training, changes in the sensitivity of diagnostic tests, and the influence of the various medical and surgical interventions on the natural history. In order best to eliminate the influence of these factors, a suitable study should (a) extend over a reasonably long period of time; (b) include a sufficiently large number of patients; (c) be carried out in a unit with a well-defined and consistent policy of diagnosis and management; (d) take account of the effect caused by the development of more specific or sensitive diagnostic tools, and (e) take account of any changes in the timing and nature of therapeutic interventions over the study period. If such criteria can be fulfilled it becomes possible to define real changes in the natural history of a disease.

The only major aspect of inflammatory bowel disease which has been studied specifically with time trends in mind is the epidemiological aspect.

A large number of studies from Europe and North America have examined the incidence and prevalence of these diseases [1].

The Incidence of Idiopathic Colitis and Its Change with Time

Despite differences in size and methodology of almost all individual studies the average annual incidence rate of idiopathic colitis varies only moderately from 3.5 per 10^5 [2] to 8.1 per 10^5 [3]. The exceptions are two studies from Britain in which the incidence rates were 11.3 per 10^5 [4] and 15.1 per 10^5 [5]. Both of these studies were remarkable for the completeness of the data collection. Although it has generally been believed that the incidence rate of idiopathic colitis has remained stable while that of Crohn's disease has risen in the last thirty years or more, several studies show an increase in incidence of idiopathic colitis [3, 4, 6, 7], while others have shown no change [5, 8–11].

The Incidence of Crohn's Disease and Its Change with Time

In contrast to the results of epidemiological studies of idiopathic colitis, the majority of studies of the epidemiology of Crohn's disease reveal a rise in incidence rate over time [3, 10, 12–19]. The only study showing no change in the incidence of Crohn's disease was that of *Devlin* et al. [5]. This evidence, collected from many centres using accepted epidemiological principles, indicates a remarkable increase in the incidence rate of Crohn's disease in the last 40 years. However, there is already some evidence that the rate of rise in some areas is slowing or has even reversed [20, 21].

A Changing Scene in the Clinical Pattern of Inflammatory Bowel Disease

As well as the accepted evidence for changes in certain aspects of the epidemiology of inflammatory bowel disease over time, is there any evidence of a change in the clinical pattern of these diseases? Many large studies have described in detail the clinical features, course, and prognosis of inflammatory bowel disease, but few have provided evidence of a changing clinical pattern of disease. Evidence of changes in mortality has been described by *Edwards and Truelove* [22].

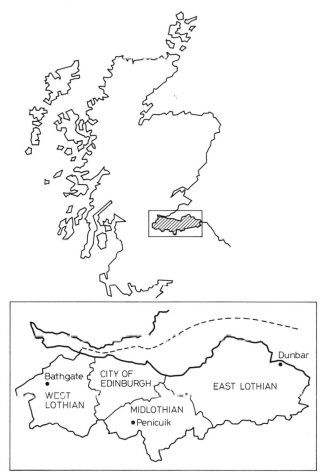

Fig. 1. Geographical location of Lothian Region.

A study by *Muscroft* et al. [23] examined the occurrence of toxic megacolon in idiopathic colitis over successive 6-year periods and revealed no difference. The extent of disease, determined in new cases presenting over time, has been studied much more in Crohn's disease [10, 14, 15, 17, 20, 24] than in idiopathic colitis [6]. In the latter study no change was found in the extent of disease. In the case of Crohn's disease the study by *Weedon* et al. [24] shows an increase in the proportion of new cases with small bowel disease and a decrease in large bowel disease, whereas those of *Miller* et al. [14] and *Kyle and Stark* [20] both show a substantial increase in the proportion of cases with large bowel disease. The studies by *Brahme* et al. [10] and *Hellers* [17] show no change in the ratio of small to large bowel disease cases with time.

Thus, while there is evidence of changes with time in certain epidemiological aspects of inflammatory bowel disease, considerably less consistent information on the clinical pattern of these diseases over time is available.

Aims and Methods

A study has been carried out which has two main aims. The first is to examine the incidence rate of idiopathic colitis and Crohn's disease in the Lothian Region of South-East Scotland during the period 1970–1979. The second is an examination of the clinical features of idiopathic colitis and Crohn's disease as seen in a gastrointestinal unit over a period of 32 years from 1950 to 1981. The aim of the study was to determine what changes may have occurred in the incidence and clinical pattern of inflammatory bowel disease over time.

Data Base for the Epidemiological Study

The geographical location of the Lothian Region is shown in figure 1. The region is the result of amalgamation of the City of Edinburgh with the counties of East-, West- and Mid-Lothian. The total population of the Region on 30th June 1979 was 750, 728 [25]. Over the study period from 1970 to 1979 the population fell by approximately 12,000, a change affecting males and females proportionately.

There were three main sources of case retrieval: (1) All in-patients and out-patients registered with the University of Edinburgh Gastrointestinal Unit at the Western General Hospital from 1970 to 1979. (2) All in-patients and out-patients registered with the Gastro-intestinal Service of the Edinburgh Royal Infirmary between 1970 and 1979. (3) A search of the computerised file of the in-patient and day case record summary sheets (SMRI) of all discharges with International Classification of Disease (ICD) codes for inflammatory bowel disease from all hospitals in the region. Care was taken to avoid counting the same patient twice.

For the epidemiological study, all patients with postal addresses outside the region were excluded as were patients diagnosed before 1970 and after 1979. In the case of Crohn's disease, patients with acute ileitis only were excluded.

Between 1970 and 1979, 807 cases of inflammatory bowel disease were identified, 498 with idiopathic colitis and 318 with Crohn's disease. The entire case notes of 478 of the 807 patients (60%) were personally scrutinised while in the remaining 329 cases reliance was placed on the diagnosis of the consultant physician or surgeon in charge of the case.

To the case notes personally scrutinised by us the following diagnostic criteria were applied:

Idiopathic colitis: At least two of the following criteria had to be met: (1) typical clinical history of disease extending over 3 months or more; (2) at least two sigmoidoscopies showing a granular mucosa with spontaneous or contact bleeding; (3) typical radiological features, and (4) typical histo-pathological features.

Crohn's disease: At least two of the following criteria had to be met: (1) a compatible clinical history; (2) radiological and/or surgical appearances of Crohn's disease, and (3) pathological features characteristic of Crohn's disease.

Data Base for the Clinical Study

The clinical study is based upon an analysis of all the cases of idiopathic colitis and Crohn's disease seen and treated in the Gastrointestinal Unit at the Western General Hospital since its inception in 1950. Between 1950 and 1981, 959 cases were treated, 659 being idiopathic colitis and 300 Crohn's disease.

The first 399 cases of idiopathic colitis, seen between 1950 and 1967, were analysed and reported [26–30]. The subsequent 260 cases of idiopathic colitis seen between 1968 and 1981 were analysed using a similar protocol to, and comparisons made with, the early series. Likewise, the study of Crohn's disease cases was divided into the same two periods 1950–1967 (129 cases) and 1968–1981 (171 cases). A standard protocol was constructed to cover the personal details of each patient including the extent of disease, the occurrence of complications such as toxic megacolon and the occurrence of extra-intestinal manifestations. The minimum criteria for the diagnosis of liver disease was the presence of two or more raised alkaline phosphatase levels in a 6 month-period in the absence of osteomalacia. Evidence for arthropathy, ankylosing spondylitis and eye disease was obtained by a detailed review of the case notes. The extent of disease, at the time of presentation, was determined wherever possible.

In order to supplement the analysis of our own cases, clinical information was obtained from all the cases of inflammatory bowel disease registered with the Gastrointestinal Service of the Royal Infirmary from 1965, when the register of its patients was started. From 1965 to 1981, 282 patients were seen by the Service, 203 being cases of idiopathic colitis and 79 of Crohn's disease.

In addition, the referral pattern of patients to our own unit of the Western General Hospital was examined with particular emphasis on the referral of seriously ill patients and those with toxic megacolon. This information was gained by a questionaire sent to all physicians and surgeons in the peripheral and district hospitals by whom patients had been referred in the period before and subsequent to 1967, the date of the first analysis.

Results

The Epidemiological Study

Incidence of Idiopathic Colitis

The number of new cases of idiopathic colitis presenting each year and the annual incidence rate are shown in table I. The mean of each couplet of years was calculated and plotted as shown in figure 2, which shows a peak in 1975 with a return to the incidence rate of the early 1970s in the late 1970s with no overall change in the incidence rate over the decade. The incidence rate per year for males and females separately is shown in table II and plotted using couplets of years in figure 3. This shows that the male and female incidence rates follow each other closely.

Incidence of Crohn's Disease

Table III shows the number of new cases of Crohn's disease each year from 1970 to 1979 and the incidence rate. This reveals an insignificant

Table I. Annual incidence rate of idiopathic colitis 1970–1979

	1970	1971	1972	1973	1974	1975	1976	1977	1978	1979	
Number of cases	45	47	51	37	63	59	47	50	46	44	total 489
Incidence rate (per 10^5 population)	5.9	6.3	6.8	4.9	8.3	7.8	6.2	6.6	6.1	5.9	overall 6.5

Mean annual incidence for 5-year periods (per 10^5 population)	1970–1974	1975–1979	p
	6.4	6.5	NS

Table II. Annual incidence rate of idiopathic colitis by gender 1970–1979

	1970	1971	1972	1973	1974	1975	1976	1977	1978	1979	
Incidence rate (male) (per 10^5 population)	4.9	4.4	6.6	5.8	8.3	8.6	7.2	6.4	4.5	7.3	overall 6.4
Incidence rate (female) (per 10^5 population)	6.8	7.8	6.7	4.0	8.3	7.1	5.3	6.8	7.6	4.6	overall 6.5

Mean annual incidence for 5-year periods (per 10^5 population)	1970–1974	1975–1979	p
Male	6.0	6.8	NS
Female	6.7	6.3	NS

Table III. Annual incidence rate of Crohn's disease 1970–1979

	1970	1971	1972	1973	1974	1975	1976	1977	1978	1979	
Number of cases	31	30	23	29	34	28	34	43	31	35	total 318
Incidence rate (per 10^5 population)	4.1	4.0	3.1	3.8	4.5	3.7	4.5	5.7	4.1	4.7	overall 4.2

	1970–1974	1975–1979	p
Mean annual incidence for 5-year periods (per 10^5 polpulation)	3.9	4.5	NS

Table IV. Annual incidence rate of Crohn's disease by gender 1970–1979

	1970	1971	1972	1973	1974	1975	1976	1977	1978	1979	
Incidence rate (male) (per 10^5 population)	4.6	3.9	1.9	2.7	2.8	2.5	3.1	5.0	2.2	2.8	overall 3.2
Incidence rate (female) (per 10^5 population)	3.5	4.0	4.0	4.7	6.0	4.8	5.8	6.3	5.9	6.4	overall 5.1

	1970–1974	1975–1979	p
Mean annual incidence for 5-year periods (per 10^5 population)			
Male	3.2	3.1	NS
Female	4.4	5.8	<0.01

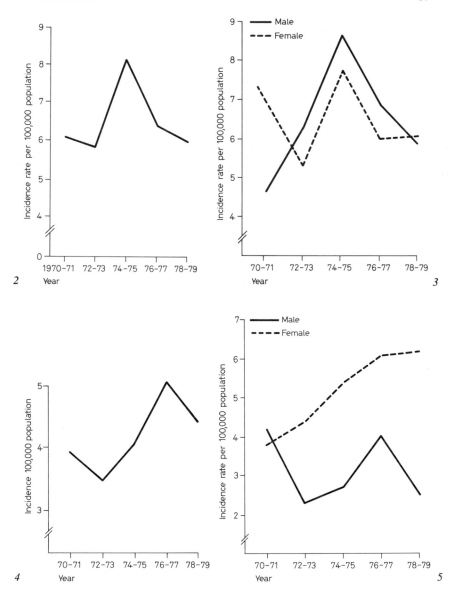

Fig. 2. Mean annual incidence of idiopathic colitis per 2 years.
Fig. 3. Incidence of idiopathic colitis by gender.
Fig. 4. Mean annual incidence of Crohn's disease per 2 years.
Fig. 5. Incidence of Crohn's disease by gender.

Table V. The incidence of toxic megacolon in idiopathic colitis

	1950–1967	1968–1981	p
Western General Hospital			
Number of cases of toxic megacolon	55	13	
Number of cases of idiopathic colitis	399	260	
% with toxic megacolon	14	5	0.01
	1968–1969	1970–1979	
Royal Infirmary			
Number of cases of toxic megacolon	3	4	
Number of cases of idiopathic colitis	23	227	
% with toxic megacolon	13	1.8	0.01

Table VI. The incidence of toxic megacolon in Crohn's disease

	1950–1967	1968–1981	p
Number of cases of toxic megacolon	2	5	
Number of cases of Crohn's disease	129	171	
% with toxic megacolon	1.6	2.9	NS

increase in mean incidence from 3.9 per 10^5 per year in the first 5 years to 4.5 per 10^5 per year in the second 5 years. The results are expressed as the mean of each couplet of years in figure 4. The incidence rate by year and gender is shown in table IV and expressed graphically in figure 5. This shows no overall change in the male incidence rate but a statistically significant rise in the incidence rate in females from 4.4 per 10^5 per year for the first 5 years to 5.8 per 10^5 per year for the second 5 years. There is no sign of a reversal of this upward trend in females towards the end of the study period.

The Clinical Study

Complications of Inflammatory Bowel Disease

Toxic Megacolon. Comparing the periods 1950–1967 and 1968–1981 at the Western General Hospital, the incidence of toxic megacolon in idiopathic colitis was found to have fallen significantly. Analysis of the Royal Infirmary data demonstrates a similar decline in this complication (table V).

The questionnaire to physicians and surgeons in peripheral hospitals who had previously regularly referred severely ill patients to the Gastro-

Table VII. Liver disease in inflammatory bowel disease

	1950–1967	1968–1981	p
Idiopathic colitis			
Number of cases of liver disease	59	11	
Number of cases of idiopathic colitis	399	260	
% with liver disease	14.8	4.2	0.001
Crohn's disease			
Number of cases of liver disease	9	11	
Number of cases of Crohn's disease	129	171	
% with liver disease	7	6.4	NS

Table VIII. Arthropathy and ankylosing spondylitis in inflammatory bowel disease

	1950–1967	1968–1981	p
Idiopathic colitis			
Cases with peripheral arthritis	27	13	
Cases of idiopathic colitis	399	260	
% with peripheral arthritis	6.7	5	NS
Cases with ankylosing spondylitis	17	5	
Cases with idiopathic colitis	399	260	
% with ankylosing spondylitis	4.3	1.9	NS
Crohn's disease			
Cases with peripheral arthritis	9	13	
Cases of Crohn's disease	129	171	
% with peripheral arthritis	7	7.6	NS
Cases with ankylosing spondylitis	6	8	
Cases of Crohn's disease	129	171	
% with ankylosing spondylitis	4.7	4.7	NS

intestinal Unit resulted in a 100% response and the universal reply that they were no longer seeing such cases.

Respecting Crohn's disease, when the two periods were compared, it was found that in contrast to the situation with idiopathic colitis, an insignificant increase in the incidence of toxic megacolon had occurred in recent years (table VI).

Liver Disease. There has been a highly significant fall in the incidence of liver disease in idiopathic colitis in recent years (table VII). A contrasting situation prevails in the case of Crohn's disease. No significant change has occurred nor is there any evidence of a declining trend (table VII).

Table IX. Eye disease in inflammatory bowel disease

	1950–1967	1968–1981	p
Idiopathic colitis			
Cases with eye disease	16	5	
Cases of idiopathic colitis	399	260	
% with eye disease	4	1.9	NS
Crohn's disease			
Cases with eye disease	2	2	
Cases with Crohn's disease	129	171	
% with eye disease	1.6	1.2	NS

Table X. Distribution of macroscopic disease in idiopathic colitis

	1950–1967		1968–1981			
Number in whom extent is known	395		241			
	Observed		Observed		Expected	p
	n	%	n	%		
Total	131	36	59	25	88	<0.01
Subtotal	149	42	73	30	100	<0.01
Distal	79	22	109	45	53	<0.001

Arthropathy and Ankylosing Spondylitis. In idiopathic colitis, the incidence of both these complications has declined in recent years but without reaching statistical significance (table VIII). No change occurred in the incidence of these complications in Crohn's disease (table VIII).

Eye Disease. In idiopathic colitis the trend was towards a reduction in the incidence of eye disease in recent years, but in Crohn's disease little change was seen (table IX).

Distribution of Macroscopic Disease

Of the 399 cases of idiopathic colitis from the pre-1967 era, the precise extent of disease was known in 359 (90%) and for ease of comparison was divided into three groups on the basis of X-ray appearance: (a) total involvement; (b) sub-total, and (c) distal, without extension above the rectosigmoid junction. In the 260 cases seen since 1967, the precise extent of disease was known in 241 (93%) and has been divided into similar

Table XI. Distribution of macroscopic lesions in Crohn's disease: frequency of area involved

	1950–1967	1968–1981		
Number of Cases	129	171		
	Observed	Observed	Expected	p
Site				
Jejunum	23	27	30	NS
Ileum	104	106	138	<0.001
Right colon	68	75	90	NS
Left colon	45	79	60	<0.05
Rectum	23	64	30	<0.001
Perineum	34	67	45	<0.02

groups to allow comparison to be made. The results are expressed in table X and show a highly significant increase in recent years in the number of new cases with disease confined to the rectum along with significant decreases in both total and sub-total disease.

The extent of macroscopic disease is known in all cases of Crohn's disease from our own unit. The sites of macroscopic disease were designated jejunum, ileum, right colon, left colon, rectum and perineum. The frequency with which each area was involved was calculated and the two eras compared (table XI). A highly significant fall has occurred in the frequency of involvement of the ileum. On the other hand, a highly significant increase in rectal disease has occurred over the same period, along with significant increases in perineal and left colonic involvement.

Discussion

The purpose of studying the epidemiology of inflammatory bowel disease is to display its natural history and to identify possible risk factors involved [1]. Several studies of the epidemiology of idiopathic colitis or Crohn's disease, or both, have been carried out in Britain [4–6, 11, 13–16, 20, 21, 31–33]. Although some have been studies from Scotland, the area of South-East Scotland has not previously been the subject of such an epidemiological study. It is of interest, therefore, that the results are similar to those derived from other centres, with the exception of the studies by *Sinclair* et al. [4] and *Devlin* et al. [5]. The absence of an overall change in the incidence of idiopathic colitis, and rise in the incidence of Crohn's disease are also compatible with the majority of previous studies.

In the case of Crohn's disease the finding of a statistically significant rise in the incidence rate in females alone, unaccompanied by any change in men, has not previously been described. However, *Kyle* [13] has remarked that a large proportion of the increased incidence of Crohn's disease which he found in North-East Scotland was due to older women with colonic disease. Such a clear distinction in the female incidence rate suggests the influence of an environmental agent affecting women more than, or rather than, men. Of the many environmental agents postulated as being involved, the only ones which affect men and women differently are the contraceptive pill and the national smoking habit: cigarette smoking has progressively increased in women in the last two decades in this country while in men the rate is falling.

The results of the clinical study showing a significant decline in the incidence of those complications associated with severe idiopathic colitis while showing no such decline in Crohn's disease, suggest either a changing population of cases of idiopathic colitis or a true decline in the severity of the disease. This is also relevant to the changing distribution of disease as, in general, the severity of idiopathic colitis is positively correlated with the extent of disease. It could be argued that as a consequence of greater awareness of the disease, a change in the referral pattern, and the use of more sensitive diagnostic tools, that a greater proportion of milder cases will be treated without there being an overall change in the severity of the disease. If this were the case one would expect the number of severely ill patients to remain constant, which the results of our questionnaire to peripheral district hospitals refutes. From the epidemiological study we have no evidence that diagnostic transfer between idiopathic colitis and Crohn's disease has occurred to any extent.

In the case of disease extent in idiopathic colitis, the finding of a greater proportion of patients with distal disease is the opposite of what would be expected if the introduction of more sensitive diagnostic tests, such as double-contrast barium enema and colonoscopy, had in themselves had any influence.

The reasons for the decline in the severity and extent of idiopathic colitis disease are unknown. It is possible that it reflects a decline in the virulence of whatever aetiological agent may be involved, or that an increase in intrinsic resistance to such an agent may have developed.

With respect to Crohn's disease there is evidence that some of the complications are related to the distribution of macroscopic disease as well as to its severity, and an increasing trend in the incidence of complications has accompanied the increasing incidence rate in contrast to the situation in idiopathic colitis. Respecting the extent of Crohn's disease, the results presented here are similar to those found in all but one of the studies previously published which have specifically examined the question of the extent of disease in new cases, over time. Undoubtedly, the increased recognition of Crohn's colitis since 1960 has played a part in this apparent shift but cannot account for it entirely. If the increase in colonic disease were the result of greater recognition of this subtype rather than a true causal shift, a significant decline in the occurrence of ileal disease at the same time would not have been expected.

The evidence presented here suggests that not only in epidemiological behaviour are changes occurring in the inflammatory bowel diseases but also in the clinical presentations and pattern of disease. This has implications for our understanding of these diseases in terms both of management and prognosis, and of aetiological and pathogenetic mechanisms.

References

1   Mendeloff, A. I.: The epidemiology of idiopathic inflammatory bowel disease; in Kirsner, Shorter, Inflammatory bowel disease; 2nd ed. (Lea & Febiger, Philadelphia 1980).

2   Garland, C. F.; Lilienfeld, A. M.; Mendeloff, A. I.; Markowitz, J. A.; Terrell, K. B.; Garland, F. C.: Incidence rates of ulcerative colitis and Crohn's disease in fifteen areas of the United States. Gastroenterology *81:* 1115–1124 (1981).

3   Binder, V.; Both, H.; Hansen, P. K.; Hendriksen, C.; Kreiner, S.; Torp-Pederson, K.: Incidence and prevalence of ulcerative colitis and Crohn's disease in the County of Copenhagen. Gastroenterology *83:* 563–568 (1982).

4   Sinclair, T. S.; Brunt, P. W.; Mowat, N. A. G.: Non-specific proctocolitis in Northeastern Scotland. A community study. Gastroenterology *85:* 1–11 (1983).

5   Devlin, H. B.; Datta, D.; Dellipiani, A. W.: The incidence and prevalence of inflammatory bowel disease in North Tees Health District. Wld J. Surg. *4:* 183–193 (1980).

6   Evans, J. G.; Acheson, E. D.: An epidemiological study of ulcerative colitis and regional enteritis in the Oxford area, Gut *6:* 311–324 (1965).

7   Sedlack, R. E.; Nobrega, F. T.; Kurland, L. T.; Sauer, W. G.: Inflammatory colon disease in Rochester, Minnesota 1935–64. Gastroenterology *62:* 935–941 (1972).

8   Bonnevie, O.; Rus, P.; Anthonisen, P.: An epidemiological study of ulcerative colitis in Copenhagen County. Scand. J. Gastroent. *9:* 81–91 (1968).

9   Myren, J.; Gjone, E.; Hertzberg, J. N.; Rygvold, O.; Semb, L. S.; Frethein, B.: Epidemiology of ulcerative colitis and regional enterocolitis (Crohn's disease) in Norway. Scand. J. Gastroent. *6:* 511–514 (1971).

10   Brahme, F.; Lindstrom, C.; Wenckert, A.: Crohn's disease in a defined population. Gastroenterology *69:* 342–351 (1975).

11   Morris, T.; Rhodes, J.: Incidence of ulcerative colitis in the Cardiff region 1968–1977. Gut *25:* 846–848 (1984).

12   Norlen, B. J.; Krause, U.; Bergman, L.: An epidemiological study of Crohn's disease. Scand. J. Gastroent. *5:* 383–390 (1970).

13   Kyle, J.: An epidemiological study of Crohn's disease in North-east Scotland. Gastroenterology *61:* 826–833 (1971).

14 Miller, D. S.; Keighley, A. C.; Langman, M. J. S.: Changing patterns in epidemiology of Crohn's disease. Lancet *ii:* 691–693 (1974).

15 Smith, I. S.; Young, S.; Gillespie, G.; O'Connor, J.; Bell, J. R.; Epidemological aspects of Crohn's disease in Clydesdale 1961 1970. Gut *16:* 62–67 (1975).

16 Mayberry, J.; Rhodes, J.; Hughes, L. E.: Incidence of Crohn's disease in Cardiff between 1934 and 1977. Gut *20:* 602–608 (1979).

17 Hellers, G.: Crohn's disease in Stockholm County 1955–1974. A study of epidemiology, results of surgical treatment and long-term prognosis. Acta chir. scand., suppl. 490, pp. 1–84 (1979).

18 Rozen, O.; Zonis, J.; Yekutiel, P.; Gilat, T.: Crohn's disease in the Jewish population of Tel-Aviv-Yafo. Gastroenterology *76:* 25–30 (1979).

19 Sedlack, R. E.; Whisnant, J.; Elveback, L. R.; Kurland, L. T.: Incidence of Crohn's disease in Olmsted County, Minnesota 1935–1975. Am. J. Epidem. *112:* 759–763 (1980).

20 Kyle, J.; Stark, G.: Fall in the incidence of Crohn's disease. Gut *21:* 340–343 (1980).

21 Harries, A. D.; Baird, A.; Rhodes, J.; Mayberry, J. F.: Has the rising incidence of Crohn's disease reached a plateau? Br. med. J. *284:* 706 (1982).

22 Edwards, F. C.; Truelove, S. C.: The course and prognosis of ulcerative colitis. Gut *4:* 299–315 (1963).

23 Muscroft, T. J.; Warren, P. M.; Asquith, P.; Montgomery, R. D.; Sokhi, G. S.: Toxic megacolon in ulcerative colitis. A continuing challenge. Post-grad. med. J. *57:* 223–227 (1981).

24 Weedon, D. D.; Shorter, R. G.; Istrup, D. M.; Huizenga, K. A.; Taylor, W. F.: Crohn's disease and cancer. New Engl. J. Med. *289:* 1099–1103 (1973).

25 Registrar General Population Statistics (IIMSO, London 1979).

26 Jalan, K. N.; Prescott, R. H.; Sircus, W.; Card, W. I.; McManus, J. P. A.; Falconer, C. W. A.; Small, W. P.; Smith, A. N.; Bruce, J.: An experience of ulcerative colitis. I. Toxic dilatation in 55 cases. Gastroenterology *57:* 68–82 (1969).

27 Jalan, K. N.; Prescott, R. J.; Walker, R. J.; Sircus, W,; McManus, J. P. A.; Card, W.: Arthropathy, ankylosing spondylitis and clubbing of fingers in ulcerative colitis. Gut *11:* 748–754 (1970).

28 Jalan, K. N.; Prescott, R. J.; Sircus, W.; Card, W. I.; McManus, J. P. A.; Falconer, C. W. A.; Small, W. P.; Smith, A. N.; Bruce, J.: An experience of ulcerative colitis. II. Short-term outcome. Gastroenterology *59:* 589–597 (1970).

29 Jalan, K. N.; Prescott, R. J.; Sircus, W.; Card, W. I.; McManus, J. P. A.; Falconer, C. W. A.; Small, W. P.; Smith, A. N.; Bruce, J.: An experience of ulcerative colitis. III. Long-term outcome. Gastroenterology *59:* 598–609 (1970).

30 Jalan, K. N.; Prescott, R. J.; Sircus, W.; Card, W. I.; McManus, J. P. A.; Falconer, C. W. A.; Small, W. P.; Smith, A. N.; Bruce, J.: Ulcerative colitis. A clinical study of 399 patients. J. R. Coll. Surg. Edinburgh *16:* 338–351 (1971).

31 Kyle, J.; Blair, D. W.: Epidemiology of regional enteritis in North-east Scotland. Br. J. Surg. *52:* 215–217 (1965).

32 Tresadern, J. C.; Gear, M. W. L.; Nicol, A.: An epidemiological study of regional enteritis in the Gloucester area. Br. J. Surg. *60:* 366–368 (1973).

33 Humphreys, W. G.; Parks, T. G.: Crohn's disease in Northern Ireland. A retrospective study of 159 cases. Irish J. med. Sci. *144:* 437–446 (1975).

Dr. W. Sircus, Consultant Physician, Gastroenterology Unit, University of Edinburgh, Western General Hospital, Edinburgh EH4 2XU (UK)

Time Trends

Front. gastrointest. Res., vol. 11, pp. 88–93 (Karger, Basel 1986)

Inflammatory Bowel Disease in Baltimore, 1960–1979: Hospital Incidence Rates, Bimodality and Smoking Factors[1]

Albert I. Mendeloff [a], *Beverly M. Calkins* [a], *Abraham M. Lilienfeld* [a], *Cedric F. Garland* [b], *Mary Monk* [a]

[a] Johns Hopkins University, School of Hygiene and Public Health, Department of Epidemiology, Baltimore, Md., USA; [b] University of California, School of Medicine, Department of Community and Family Medicine, San Diego, Calif., USA

Introduction

The first study of the incidence rates for inflammatory bowel diseases (IBD) in the metropolitan area of Baltimore, Md. was carried out in 1960–1963 [1]. The investigators responsible for that study have continued to be interested in the subject, and have repeated the investigation of IBD incidence in 1973 and 1977–1979. This report summarizes the findings of the three surveys and discusses trends in incidence, the bimodality of the age distribution and the relationship of smoking to IBD. The size of the population at risk has not changed appreciably over the 20 years, and has been carefully monitored by census appraisers in 1970 and 1980. It is important to realize, however, that the incidence rates are based entirely on *first hospitalization* data. If changes in medical practice over this period have resulted in different rates of hospitalizing patients suspected of having IBD, the rates the authors report may well reflect such changes. No information is available regarding the magnitude or importance of these changes, and therefore the findings will simply represent first hospitalization rates.

[1] Supported in part by Grants No. AM 18021 and AM 20467 from the National Institute of Arthritis, Metabolism and Digestive Diseases. Dr. *Calkins* is a recipient of a Research Career Award from the National Foundation for Ileitis and Colitis, Inc. Dr. *Lilienfeld* is a recipient of Research Career Award No. K06-GM 13901 from the National Institute of General Medical Sciences.

Methods

The approach used to ascertain *incident cases* from admissions at each of the 24 hospitals in the Baltimore Standard Metropolitan Statistical Area (SMSA) was similar in each of the surveys [1, 2]. Cases consisted of hospital admissions chosen from the diagnostic index of admitted patients. A list was developed of potential study cases who were diagnosed as having diseases including the following ICD categories: (ICD-9) regional enteritis (555), idiopathic proctocolitis (556), irritable colon (564.10), ulcer of anus and rectum (569.41); (ICD-8) chronic enteritis and ulcerative colitis (563) and other diseases of intestines and peritoneum (569); and (H-ICDA) chronic enteritis and ulcerative colitis (563) and other diseases of intestines and peritoneum (569). Information from the hospital records of these potential cases was abstracted to determine their eligibility for study and their demographic characteristics. Potential cases were excluded if the record indicated that the patient had been treated for the conditions of interest prior to the beginning of the study period, or if the diagnostic information was not sufficient or if the patient's residence at the time of admission was outside the Baltimore SMSA. Each incident case was assigned a diagnosis based on recorded information and an estimated degree of certainty of diagnosis (definite, probable, possible) by the same gastroenterologist (*A.I.M.*), in all three studies, using the diagnostic criteria presented in previous reports [1, 2]. Definite and probable cases were combined and this group was defined as cases.

Age-adjusted rates using the 1970 Baltimore SMSA census population as a standard were calculated for both color and sex groups to determine trends for the combined group of definite and probable cases. Cases of ulcerative colitis (UC) and ulcerative proctitis were grouped together. Cases of Crohn's disease (CD) with and without mention of colonic involvement were also grouped together for these calculations. The adjusted rates were limited to age groups over 20 years of age to permit comparisons with the 1960–1963 data which were confined to these age groups. Confidence intervals for the age-adjusted rates were calculated according to the method suggested by *Lilienfeld and Lilienfeld* [3]. The age and sex distributions of the populations ascertained in the 1960, 1970, and 1980 censuses were used to calculate age-specific rates. Data on age-specific rates presented here are limited to whites. The rates for non-whites have been presented elsewhere but they are based on numbers too small for any assessment of age-specific trends or even modality of the age-specific distribution [4].

Bimodality was evaluated by visually examining the graphs of the age-specific distributions and by calculating a ratio of the first peak rate to that of the first trough and of the second peak to the first trough with the use of the numerical values of the age-specific rates. A ratio of peak to trough equal to or greater than 1.50 for peaks on *both sides* of the trough, which indicates an increased risk of 50 per cent or greater of both peak decades over the trough decade, was arbitrarily set as providing a criterion for bimodality. Finally, the relationship of smoking to both UC and CD was evaluated in the 1977–1979 survey [5] by comparing cases and controls using both unmatched and paired analysis.

Results

Trends of age-adjusted rates per 100,000 population during 1960–1979 for definite and probable cases for white and nonwhite males and females for UC and CD are shown in figures 1 and 2, respectively.

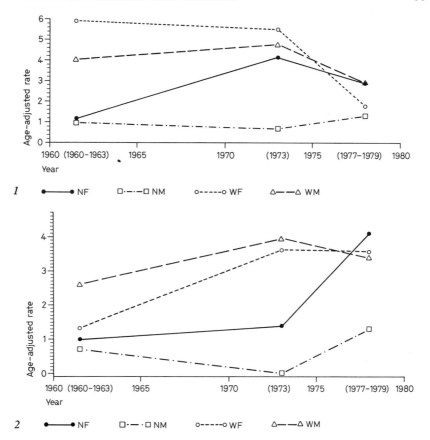

Fig. 1. Trends in the average annual age-adjusted incidence rates (per 100,000) of ulcerative colitis in Baltimore, 1960–1979. Rates adjusted to the 1970 census population using 20+ age categories only. WM = white males; WF = white females; NM = non-white males; NF = non-white females.

Fig. 2. Trends in the average annual age-adjusted incidence rates (per 100,000) of Crohn's disease in Baltimore, 1960–1979. Rates adjusted to the 1970 census population using 20+ age categories only. WM = white males; WF = white females; NM = non-white males; NF = non-white females.

Among whites for both sexes, the rates were fairly stable for UC between 1960–1963 and 1973 but declined markedly between 1973 and 1977–1979. For non-white females rates increased between 1960–1963 and 1973, followed by a decline to 1977–1979. The rates for non-white males appear to be consistently low and relatively unchanged. In contrast to UC, the rates for CD for whites consistently increased between 1960–

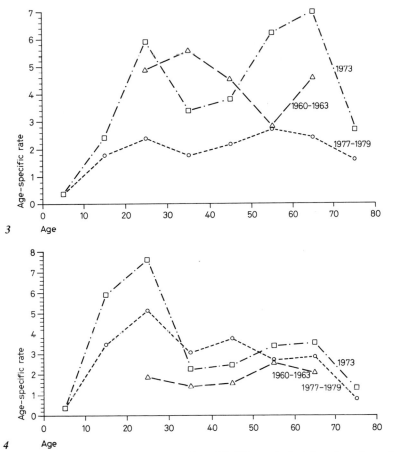

Fig. 3. Age-specific incidence rates (per 100,000 population) for ulcerative colitis in Baltimore, 1960–1979 for whites.

Fig. 4. Age-specific incidence rates (per 100,000 population) for Crohn's disease in Baltimore, 1960–1979 for whites.

1963 and 1973 and then stabilized between 1973 and 1977–1979. Non-white female rates increased slightly between 1960–1963 and 1973, whereas non-white male rates declined slightly. Non-white rates for both sexes increased sharply between 1973 and 1977–1979.

The *age-specific rates* per 100,000 population in 1960–1979 for definite and probable cases for white males and females for UC and CD are shown in figures 3 and 4, respectively. Because of the relatively small numbers of cases in each age category, trends over time for specific ages are difficult to interpret.

The rather arbitrary criterion for *bimodality* is met by all three Baltimore surveys of definite and probable UC cases. The first peak occurs in age group 30–39 in the 1960–1963 survey and at 20–29 years in the two recent surveys. The second peak occurs in the age group 60–69 in the first two surveys and somewhat earlier, 50–59 years, in the last survey. A pattern of bimodality is evident in the age distributions for CD, but is less distinctive than for UC and only marginally meets the criteria for bimodality.

In assessing an association with *smoking* in the 1977–1979 survey, the only consistent finding was a higher frequency of non-smokers among UC cases compared to the hospital control group among males; this association was found in both matched and unmatched analyses. Among UC male cases compared with neighborhood controls, the association was found in the matched analysis, which controlled to some extent for socioeconomic level status of the groups. A higher frequency of smokers was found among CD cases when compared with neighborhood controls among males and both sexes combined, in an unmatched analysis. However, differences disappeared in matched analysis, when socioeconomic level was controlled.

Discussion

In Baltimore the age-adjusted rates for CD have increased from 1960 to 1979 to exceed those for UC among whites of both sexes and non-white females whereas rates for UC have declined. The UC and CD rates for non-white males are similar. The rates for white males exceed those for non-white males for both UC and CD, but the converse is true for females. In 1977–1979 females have higher rates than males for CD in both color groups and for UC among non-whites, while white UC rates are higher for males than for females. From the first to the second surveys, the white male and female rates for UC converge with increasing male and decreasing female rates, but then both decline from the second to the third surveys. For CD, the age-adjusted rates increased from the first to second surveys for whites of both sexes and for non-white females. The CD rates appeared to stabilize for whites of both sexes between the second and third surveys, but they increased for non-whites of both sexes.

Greater familiarity among physicians with mild UC may have resulted in fewer hospitalizations in 1977–1979 than in the previous surveys, but it is not possible to answer this question definitely. For CD, rates have increased from 1960–1979, with the highest rates in 1973 for whites and in 1977–1979 for non-whites.

In the 1960–1963 study, subjects less than 20 years of age were excluded. However, in 1973 and 1977–1979, when this group was included, it was found that incident cases under age 20 were plentiful, with rates similar to or higher than those of ages 30–39 and 40–49. Rates for UC in those over 60 are also relatively high, definitely supporting a bimodal incidence. Bimodality has been a consistent feature of UC in Baltimore but is not as prominent for the most recent survey of CD.

The higher frequency of non-smokers among UC cases reported by others in 1982–1984 [6–11] was found in this survey only in males when compared to hospital controls and to matched neighborhood controls. It must be emphasized that the other reported studies included both prevalent and incident cases whereas the Baltimore study was limited to incident cases which are more appropriate for the investigation of such relationships. Additional studies of such associations are needed before definitive conclusions can be inferred.

References

1   Monk, M.; Mendeloff, A. I.; Siegel, C. I.; Lilienfeld, A. M.: An epidemiological study of ulcerative colitis and regional enteritis among adults in Baltimore. I. Hospital incidence and prevalence, 1960 to 1963. Gastroenterology 53: 198–210 (1967).
2   Garland, C. F.; Lilienfeld, A. M.; Mendeloff, A. L.; Markowitz, J. A.; Terrell, K. B.; Garland, F. C.: Trend in incidence rates of ulcerative colitis and Crohn's disease in Baltimore (in preparation)
3   Lilienfeld, A. M.; Lilienfeld, D. E.: Foundations of epidemiology; 2nd ed., p. 358 (Oxford University Press, New York 1980).
4   Calkins, B. M.; Lilienfeld, A. M.; Mendeloff, A. I.; Gerland, C. F.: Trend in the incidence of ulcerative colitis and CD. Dig. Dis. Sci. (in press).
5   Calkins, B. M.; Lilienfeld, A. M.; Mendeloff, A. I.; Gerland, C. F.; Monk, M.: Smoking factors in ulcerative colitis and Crohn's disease in Baltimore. Proc. Soc. epidem. Res., Houston 1984.
6   Jick, H.; Walker, A. M.: Cigarette smoking and ulcerative colitis. New Engl. J. Med. 308: 261–263 (1983).
7   Harries, A. D.; Baird, A.; Rhodes, J.: Non-smoking. A feature of ulcerative colitis. Br. med. J. 284: 706 (1982).
8   Bures, J.; Fixa, B.; Komarkova, O.; Fingerland, A.: Letter. Br. med. J. 285: 440 (1982).
9   Logan, R. F. A.; Edmond, M.; Somerville, K. W.; Langman, M. J. S.: Smoking and ulcerative colitis. Br. med. J. 288: 751–753 (1984).
10 Gyde, S. N.; Prior, P.; Taylor, K.; Allan, R. N.: Cigarette smoking, blood pressure, and ulcerative colitis (Abstract). Gut 24: A998 (1983).
11 Penny, W. J.; Penny, E.; Mayberry, J. F.; Rhodes, J.: Mormons, smoking and ulcerative colitis. Lancet ii: 1315 (1983).

Dr. Albert I. Mendeloff, Department of Epidemiology, School of Hygiene and Public Health, Johns Hopkins University, 615 N. Wolfe, Baltimore, MD 21205 (USA)

Front. gastrointest. Res., vol. 11, pp. 94–101 (Karger, Basel 1986)

Crohn's Disease in Galicia, Spain. – 1968–1982

V. Ruiz, J. Potel

University Hospital, Santiago de Compostela, Spain

Crohn's disease (CD) was very rarely found in Spain 20 years ago when many of the countries of North-Western Europe and North America reported an incidence of about 1.5 new cases per year per 100,000 inhabitants [1–6].

Galicia is a region situated in the north-west of Spain. It borders on the north and west with the Atlantic Ocean and in the south with Portugal (fig. 1). Its area is 29,434 km² (5.8% of Spain), divided into four provinces, having a moderate and wet Atlantic climate. It has a relatively stable population of 2,725,000 inhabitants. There are eight General Hospitals, a University School of Medicine and a Society of Gastroenterology. All these factors make Galicia particularly suitable for epidemiological studies.

In 1976 the Galician Society of Gastroenterology prepared the first epidemiological study of CD in Galicia and we found only 39 cases in the period from 1966 to 1975. This gave an annual incidence of 0.14/100,000, approximately a tenth of the incidence in the northern European countries [7]. Seven years later, in 1983, we made a new epidemiological survey. The results are presented and compared to the first study.

Material and Methods

The survey method used was based on a questionnaire describing the most relevant features of each patient. This was sent to all members of the Galician Society of Gastroenterology and to all the hospitals of the region.

In order to be included in this study, each patient had to meet at least two of the four following diagnostic criteria [2]: (1) clinical features – diarrhea, abdominal colic, weight loss; (2) macroscopic appearances of CD at operation or necropsy; (3) microscopic features of CD in biopsy or resected specimens; (4) radiological features characteristic of CD.

A total of 173 answers were received from all over the region. Although we also analyzed the diagnostic, pathological and therapeutic data, the present report is concerned mainly with the results related to CD epidemiology. We used the data of definitive diagnosis for calculating disease incidence.

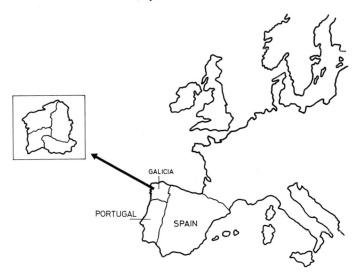

Fig. 1. Galicia is situated in the north-west corner of the Iberian Peninsula to the north of Portugal and is administratively divided into four provinces.

Results

During the 7-year study period, out of the 173 cases analyzed, 152 patients met the diagnostic criteria for inclusion in the study. The absolute number of cases per year during the study period is shown in figure 2.

The disease was more frequent in men (95) than in women (57), and the male/female ratio was 1:0.6. Compared with the expected male/female ratio in Galicia (1:1.08), the difference is significant (p < 0.01) (fig. 3).

Figure 4 shows the annual number of new cases per 100,000 population. The incidence of CD has increased from 0.52, in 1976, to 1.13 in 1982; the average was 0.8.

The incidence by age and sex was also calculated for 10-year periods (fig. 5). The peak incidence in men was between the ages 20 and 29 years and gradually decreased during the following years. In women the incidence peaked a decade later and then remained low.

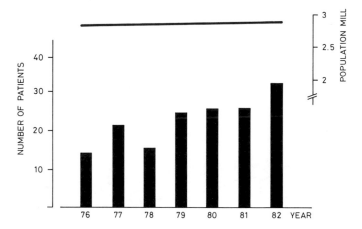

Fig. 2. The absolute number of cases of Crohn's disease in Galicia between 1976 and 1982. The population of the region during the same period of time remained almost constant.

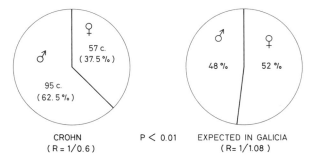

Fig. 3. Sex incidence.

The distribution of the patients with CD, within the four provinces is shown in figure 6. The four places where we found the highest incidence are sea ports, and three of them are the most industrialised and populated towns in Galicia. Yet, in Galicia, only one-third of the population reside in urban areas. Thus, the incidence is high, 1.68 per 100,000 urban population, in comparison with rural areas, 0.38, and the difference is statistically significant ($p < 0.01$) (table I).

Regarding the family history of CD, 8 cases were found amongst siblings, which represent a 5.26% incidence.

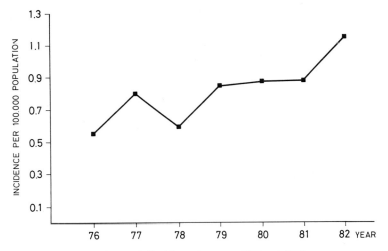

Fig. 4. Changes in the yearly incidence between 1976 and 1982.

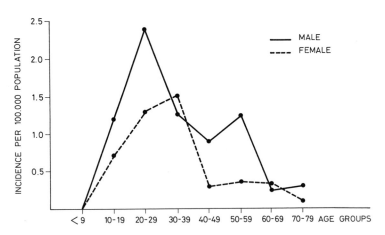

Fig. 5. Incidence in different age groups, by sex.

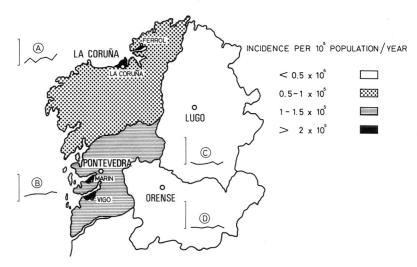

Fig. 6. Geographic distribution of CD in the different provincial areas of Galicia and the evolution of the yearly incidence of the disease in these provinces (A, B, C, D). There is an increasing trend in A and B and none in C, and D.

Table I. Place of residence: numbers of cases and rates in city and in rural areas (rates per 100,000 per year)

	Male		Female		Both sexes	
	n	rate	n	rate	n	rate
City	66	2.24	36	1.13	102	1.68
Rural	29	0.46	21	0.31	50	0.38
City + rural	95	1.03	57	0.57	152	0.80

The most frequent localization of the disease in our patients was in the small bowel only (51.3%), followed by small and large bowel (34.2%), colon and rectum (11.2%) and other areas (3.3%) (fig. 7).

The two epidemiological studies were combined so as to have perspective of 15 years, divided into 3-year periods (fig. 8). The incidence rose abruptly from 1974. The average annual incidence during the 15 years was 0.46 per 100,000 population, however if we compare the first 3-year period with the last, the incidence has risen 16-fold.

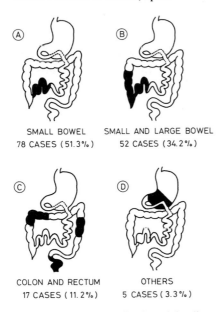

SMALL BOWEL   SMALL AND LARGE BOWEL
78 CASES (51.3%)   52 CASES (34.2%)

COLON AND RECTUM   OTHERS
17 CASES (11.2%)   5 CASES (3.3%)

Fig. 7. Anatomical localization of the disease in 152 patients.

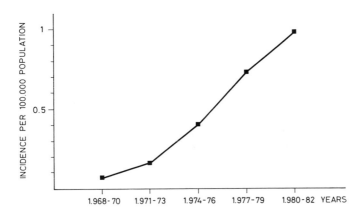

Fig. 8. Evolution of the incidence of Crohn's disease, over five 3-year periods.

Discussion

Our results confirm that the incidence of Crohn's disease in Galicia has been rising steadily from 0.14/100,000, in the former study (1966–1975) [7] to 0.8 in this study (1976–1982). However, it is still less than that recorded in the Scandinavian countries, United Kingdom and Israel [6, 8–11] during similar periods of time.

The average annual incidence during the 15 years covered by the two studies was 0.46 per 100,000 population, which is similar to that found in the other two Spanish multicenter studies [12, 13]. So, we can take this average as being representative of CD in Spain.

The age of the highest incidence was between 20 and 29 years, as found in previous studies [14]. Though the sex ratio in CD is usually equal [14], we have found a predominance in males.

In previous CD studies there has been no clear predominance among city dwellers as compared to the rural population, possibly because these epidemiological surveys were based on major urban centers [14]. However, our study is representative of the whole of the Galician region where only a third of the population live in urban areas (towns with more than 50,000 inhabitants). We have been able to clearly demonstrate the higher incidence in the urban areas. As to the geographical distribution, the incidence was highest and steadily increasing in the two predominantly coastal provinces, where the most industrialised towns are found. However, in the interior provinces, which are mainly dedicated to agriculture and cattle rearing, the incidence was continuously low.

Thus, we can say that the incidence of Crohn's disease in Galicia is very much related to the degree of industrialization in the region and is rising.

Acknowledgements

We gratefully acknowledge the following hospitals and colleagues that participated in this cooperative study: Hospital Universitario (General de Galicia), Santiago de Compostela (*R. Conde, R. Mosquera, J. Potel, J. L. Puente*); Ciudad Sanitaria Juan Canalejo, La Coruña (*F. Arnal, M. De Juan, J. Machuca, S. Pereira, H. Rodriguez, J. L. Vazquez*); Hospital de la Marina, El Ferrol (*A. Rey*); Residencia Sanitaria Arquitecto Marcide, El Ferrol (*C. Garcia-Pintos*); Hospital Provincial de Pontevedra (*M. Castro-Rial, M. A. Piñón*); POVISA, Vigo (*J. Estevez, J. Mosquera, F. Peralta*); Hospital Xeral de Vigo (*P. Blanco, J. R. Fernández-Larrañaga, R. Diaz-Ureña, M. Ferrández, P. Gil, P. Mardomingo, E. Novoa, A. Pallarés, C. Sobrino*); Residencia Sanitaria Hermanos Pedrosa, Lugo (*M. J. Alfonso, U. Romero, A. Pérez-Carnero*); Residencia Sanitaria Ntra. Sra. del Cristal, Orense (*O. Fernández, M. Vega, R. Vila*); *L. Baltar* (Santiago), *M. Carballal* (Pontevedra),

J. Fernández (Orense), R. González-Abraldes (Santiago), J. Iglesias (Santiago), G. Martin-Arribas (Vigo), D. Portela (Vigo), J. Pérez-Villanueva (Vigo), V. Ruiz (Vigo) and J. Varela (Santiago).

References

1   Monk, M.; Mendeloff, A.; Siegel, C.; Lilienfeld, A.: An epidemiological study of ulcerative colitis and regional enteritis among adults in Baltimore. I. Hospital incidence and prevalence, 1960–1963. Gastroenterology 53: 198–210 (1967).
2   Kyle, J.: An epidemiological study of Crohn's disease in Northeast Scotland. Gastroenterology 61: 826–833 (1971).
3   Fahrländer, H.; Baerlocher, C.: Clinical features and epidemiological data on Crohn's diease in the Basle area. Scand. J. Gastroent. 6: 657–662 (1971).
4   Miller, D.; Keighley A.; Langman, M.: Changing patterns in epidemiology of Crohn's disease. Lancet ii: 691–693 (1974).
5   Hellers, G.: Crohn's disease in Stockholm county, 1955–1974. Acta chir. scand. 490: suppl. (1979).
6   Mayberry, J.; Rhodes, J. Hughes; L.: Incidence of Crohn's disease in Cardiff between 1934 and 1977. Gut 20: 602–608 (1979).
7   Marina Fiol, C.; Ruiz Ochoa, V.; Portela Pérez, D.; Gonzalez Abraldes, R.; Potel Lesquereux, J.; Pérez Villanueva, J.: Simposio sobre la Enfermedad de Crohn en Galicia. Rev. Esp. Enf. Ap. Digest. 50. 469–482 (1977).
8   Kyle, J.; Stark, G.: Fall in the incidence of Crohn's disease. Gut 21: 340–343 (1980).
9   Hellers, G.: Epidemiology of Crohn's disease; in Jewell, Emanoel Lee, Topics in gastroenterology, vol. 9, pp. 13–20 (Blackwell, Oxford 1981).
10 Binder, V.; Both, H.; Hansen, P.; Hendriksen, C.; Kreiner, S.; Torp-Pedersen, K.: Incidence and prevalence of ulcerative colitis and Crohn's disease in the county of copenhagen, 1962 to 1978. Gastroenterology 83: 563–568 (1982).
11 Rozen, P.; Zonis, J.; Yekutiel, P.; Gilat, T.: Crohn's Disease in the Jewish population of Tel-Aviv-Jafo. Epidemiological and clinical aspects. Gastroenterology 76: 25–30 (1979).
12 Garcia Paredes, J.; Pajares Garcia, J.: Crohn's disease in the central area of Spain; in Peña, Weterman, Strober, Proc. 2nd Int. Workshop on Crohn's Disease, Leiden 1980. Recent advances in Crohn's disease, pp. 168–173 (Martinus Nijhoff, The Hague 1981).
13 Martinez, G.; Fernández, Y.; Rodrigo Saez, L.; Martinez, E.: Estudio epidemiologico de la enfermedad de Crohn en la región Asturiana. Rev. Esp. Enf. Ap. Digest. 63: 534–541 (1983).
14 Langman, M.; Burnham, W.: Epidemiology of inflammatory bowel disease; in Allan, Keighley, Alexander-Williams, Hawkins. Inflammatory bowel disease; 1st ed., pp. 17–23 (Churchill Livingstone, Edinburgh 1983).

Dr. V. Ruiz, Calle Dr. Cadaval, 6, Vigo 2 (Spain)

Front. gastrointest. Res., vol. 11, pp. 102–113 (Karger, Basel 1986)

The Changing Incidence of Crohn's Disease in Blackpool 1969–1983

Frank I. Lee, Francis T. Costello

Department of Gastroenterology, Victoria Hospital, Blackpool, Lancashire, UK

Introduction

The aetiology of Crohn's disease is not known. There is evidence that genetic factors may be important [1–4]. In addition, differences between geographical areas and changes in incidence and prevalence over a period of time suggest that environmental factors may make their impact on susceptible populations. There have been indications that Crohn's disease has increased in the United Kingdom since the 1960s [5–9] and a report from Blackpool has confirmed this trend in a report describing findings from 1968 to 1980 [10].

In this chapter we review the experience in Blackpool from 1969 to 1983. Blackpool is a seaside town on the Lancashire coast in North-West England (fig. 1). The main hospital is Victoria Hospital and serves the inhabitants of the Blackpool, Wyre and Fylde Health District. This population has remained at approximately 300,000 throughout the period of study. Blackpool is the main town having 170,000 inhabitants, the remainder of the area consists of small towns, namely, Fleetwood, Thornton Cleveleys, Poulton-le-Fylde, Lytham St. Annes and Kirkham. So, the population is almost entirely urban. During the period of study, there was a predominance of women in the population in a proportion of 1.12:1.

Case identification and categorization have been carried out as follows: (a) Review of patients classified in the Department of Gastroenterology Case Index as having ulcerative colitis or Crohn's disease. (b) Review of cases classified in the Department of Histopathology as having Crohn's disease in the relevant years. (c) Clinical colleagues allowed access to information about their patients. (d) The North-West Regional Health Authority, based in Manchester, gives data relating to Hospital Activity Analysis and cases classified as having Crohn's disease have been reviewed.

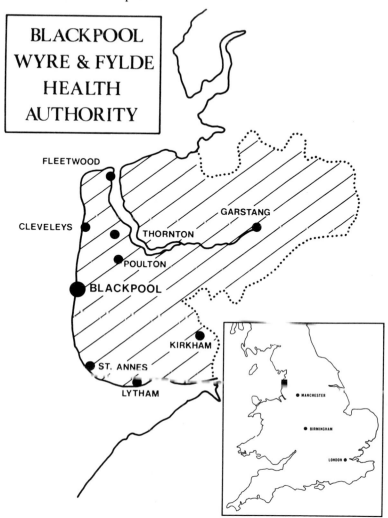

Fig. 1. Blackpool Wyre & Fylde health authority.

In this report we have analysed patients according to the year and age at which they presented for hospital assessment so that variations associated with onset-to-diagnosis delays are minimized. In some patients initially diagnosed as having ulcerative colitis, it became apparent later that Crohn's disease is the correct diagnosis. The evidence has been reassessed relating to clinical features, macroscopic appearances and histological

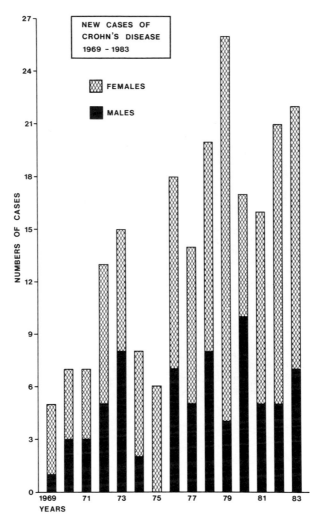

Fig. 2. New cases of Crohn's disease 1969–1983.

features of material obtained at autopsy, laparotomy and endoscopy, and typical radiological features and the diagnosis of Crohn's disease verified or refuted. Particular care was taken in reviewing cases of acute ileitis and proctitis and the possibility of ischaemic colitis was considered, particularly in the elderly. Clear descriptions of Crohn's colitis predated the period of this study [11, 12]. In addition, each case record and available

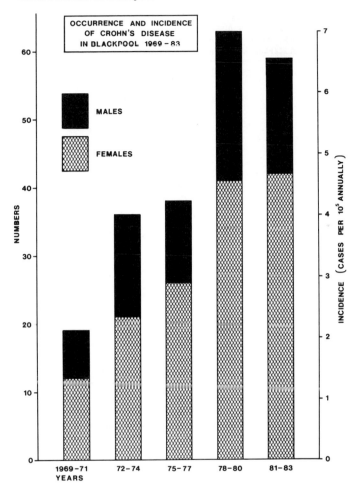

Fig. 3. Occurrence and incidence of Crohn's disease in Blackpool 1969–1983.

pathological material were reviewed retrospectively according to similar criteria. It is not likely, therefore, that increased recognition of Crohn's colitis contributed to bias in our findings.

Results

Two hundred and fifteen patients have been recognized who presented with Crohn's disease during the 15-year period 1969–1983, an *inci-*

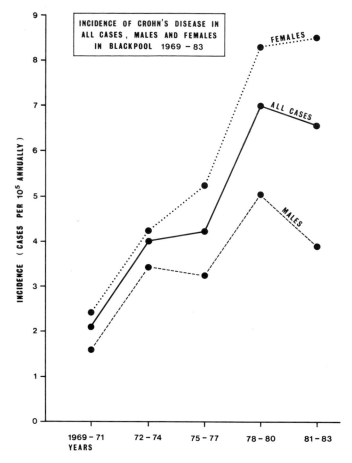

Fig. 4. Incidence of Crohn's disease in all cases, males and females, in Blackpool 1969–1983.

dence of 4.8 per 10⁵. The peak year was 1979 when the incidence was 8.7
per 10⁵ (fig. 2). There was an increase over the years of the study initially,
but levelling out occurred around 1978. On the evidence of three-yearly
figures, a plateau has been reached at the present time (fig. 3). The increase in incidence over the years is most prominent in *females*, the sex
ratio increasing from 1.7:1 in 1969–1971 to 2.5:1 in 1981–1983. The incidence increased 2.4 times in men and 3.5 times in women over the same
period of time (fig. 4). As in most other series, we have noted an approximately equal incidence of the three *anatomical types*. The overall sex
ratio was 1.95:1, highest for large bowel disease – 2.33:1 (table I). As far

Table I. Crohn's disease in Blackpool (1969–1983): Distribution of cases by sex and anatomical site

	Number	%	Female	Male	Ratio
Small bowel	78	36.2	49	29	1.69:1
Mixed	57	26.5	38	19	2.00:1
Large bowel	80	37.2	56	24	2.33:1
All cases	215	100	143	72	1.95:1

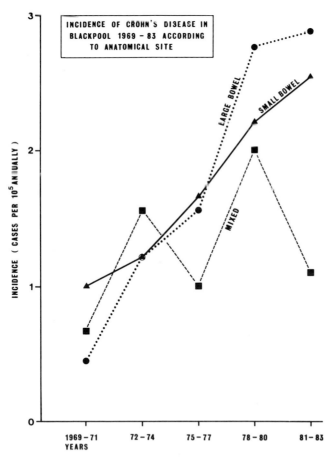

Fig. 5. Incidence of Crohn's disease in Blackpool 1969–1983 according to anatomical site.

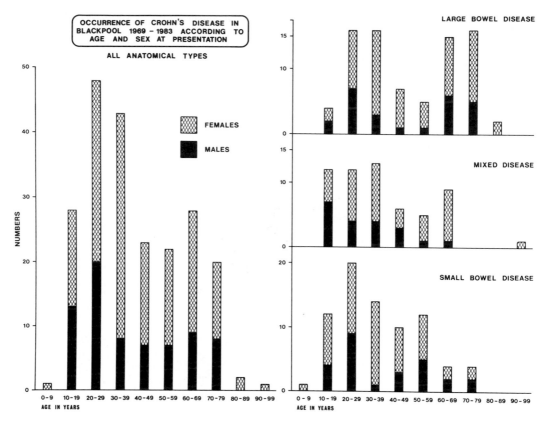

Fig. 6. Occurrence of Crohn's disease in Blackpool 1969–1983 according to age and sex at presentation. All anatomical types.

as site of disease at onset is concerned, there have been increases in purely small bowel and large bowel disease, the change in incidence being inapparent in those with mixed disease. The increase in small and large bowel disease is constant through the period being 2.5 times for small bowel and 6 times for large bowel cases (fig. 5) the change being most prominent in women. Analysis of age at presentation according to anatomical site shows a predominantly unimodal distribution for small bowel and for mixed disease with a peak in the third and fourth decades. Large bowel Crohn's disease shows a bimodal age distribution with peaks in the third and eighth decades (fig. 6).

Table II. Numbers (*a*) and incidence (*b*) per 10^5 of patients presenting with Crohn's disease according to three age ranges between 1969 and 1983 (totals and for each sex)

	10–29 years			30–54 years			55 years and above		
	male	female	total	male	female	total	male	female	total
a									
1969–1971	2	3	5	4	5	9	1	4	5
1972–1974	6	9	15	4	9	13	5	3	8
1975–1977	10	4	14	0	12	12	2	10	12
1978–1980	10	12	22	5	14	19	7	15	22
1981–1983	6	10	16	5	19	24	6	13	19
b									
1969–1971	1.62	2.49	2.04	2.97	3.57	3.28	0.76	2.12	1.55
1972–1974	4.85	7.47	6.13	2.97	3.57	4.73	3.78	1.56	2.48
1975–1977	8.10	3.32	5.72	0	8.58	4.37	1.51	5.31	3.73
1978–1980	8.10	9.95	9.00	3.71	10.01	6.92	5.31	7.96	6.83
1981–1983	4.85	8.50	6.54	3.71	13.58	8.74	4.55	6.90	5.90

Note the high incidence in females in the later years of the study in the age range 30–54 years.

Table III. Numbers (*a*) and incidence (*b*) per 10^5 of patients presenting with each anatomical type of Crohn's disease between 1969 and 1983 according to three age ranges

	10–29 years			30–54 years			55 years and above		
	SB	LB	mixed	SB	LB	mixed	SB	LB	mixed
a									
1969–1971	5	0	0	3	1	5	1	3	1
1972–1974	6	3	6	4	2	7	1	6	1
1975–1977	5	3	6	7	4	1	3	7	2
1978–1980	6	8	8	10	5	4	4	12	6
1981–1983	8	6	2	9	11	4	6	9	4
b									
1969–1971	2.04	0	0	1.09	0.36	1.82	0.31	0.93	0.31
1972–1974	2.45	1.23	2.45	1.46	0.72	2.55	0.31	1.86	0.31
1975–1977	2.04	1.23	2.45	2.55	1.46	0.36	0.93	2.17	0.62
1978–1980	2.45	3.37	3.27	3.64	1.82	1.46	1.24	3.73	1.86
1981–1983	3.27	2.45	0.82	3.28	4.01	1.46	1.86	2.80	1.24

SB = Small bowel; LB = large bowel.
Note the increase over the years and the high incidence in the later years in large bowel disease in the middle and older age groups.

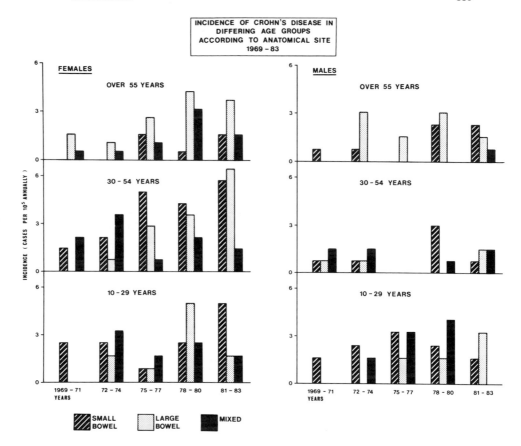

Fig. 7. Incidence of Crohn's disease in differing age groups according to anatomical site 1969–1983.

We have attempted to identify *trends* over the 15-year period with regard to the incidence of disease in three age groups 10–29, 30–54 and 55 years and above. This analysis shows a most emphatic finding – a very high incidence in the later years within the middle age range (30–54 years) in women. There was no comparable increase in this age range in men. Less marked increases in incidence in females can be shown in the younger and older age groups and also in men (table II). Table III shows changing incidence of different anatomical types of Crohn's disease according to the three age groups. Detailed analysis of the trends shows that the increase in women in the range 30–54 years is due entirely to increases in small bowel and large bowel disease. Changes in incidence of mixed disease are minor over all age ranges in men and women (fig. 7).

Discussion

The evidence from this series, based on findings in a circumscribed population in the North-West of England, suggests that there was an upward trend in the incidence of Crohn's disease until the mid-1970s. Subsequently, there has been a levelling off beginning around 1978 continuing through to 1983. The Cardiff group could find no evidence of a plateau effect up to 1980 [13]. We have previously drawn attention to an apparent fall in incidence in the mid-1970s in Blackpool [10] and suggest that this may be artefactual associated with the relative rarity of this disease and variations in onset-to-diagnosis intervals. Similar falls have also been observed in North-East Scotland [14] and Copenhagen [15] and until understanding of the condition is more complete, these observations should not be discounted. Most series have shown an approximately equal sex incidence. A few show female predominance but none as high as in the Blackpool series – overall 1.95:1. In addition, this predominance increases through the years of observation, the increase being partly accounted for by a slight fall in incidence in males towards the end of the period of study. Recent studies have shown proportions of male:female of 1:1.5 in Spokane, Washington [16], 1:1.1 in Malmo [17], and an equal sex incidence in Olmsted County, Minnesota [18]. Although the overall sex incidence in Cardiff from 1934–1977 was 1:1.4, *Mayberry* et al. [7] noted that in the last 7 years of their study, the sex difference was lost with a slight preponderance in males. Most studies show a relatively even distribution between the site of disease and this study conforms in this respect. In Blackpool an apparent diminution in the occurrence of ileocaecal disease has been noted over the years of study for women and, in particular, men. Surprisingly, no male with purely ileocaecal disease presented below the age of 30 years in 1981–1983. A diminution in the occurrence of ileocaecal disease in recent years has also been suggested in North-East Scotland [14]. However, in Cardiff in 1980, increasing incidence involving all anatomical types appeared to be continuing [13]. The later years of our study showed the highest incidence of Crohn's disease to be occurring in the middle age range (30–54 years) involving small bowel and large bowel disease. In contrast, in Minnesota the highest incidence occurred in the 20- to 29-year range in the later years (1965–1975) [18].

Interpretation of these findings must await clearer understanding of the pathogenesis of the condition. However, some speculation is in order. As yet no clear-cut conclusions have come from review of the epidemiological evidence in Crohn's disease [19–21], but clearly there are genetic and environmental factors involved. Variations between populations may relate to differing genetic backgrounds and variations in relevant environmental factors. In time, assuming that the relevant environmental factors in a given area reach a steady level, all genetically susceptible individuals within a population will become exposed so that a steady incidence may be achieved. Correspondingly, a reduction in the environmental factors may be followed by a reduction in incidence; and it may be that Crohn's disease will join other conditions whose occurrence has diminished before their pathogenesis has been clearly understood.

References

1   Mendeloff, A. I.; Monk, M.; Siegal, C. I.; Lilienfeld, A.: Some epidemiological features of ulcerative colitis and regional enteritis. A preliminary report. Gastroenterology 51: 748–756 (1966).

2   Lewkonia, R. M.; McConnell, R. B.: Familial inflammatory bowel disease. Hereditary or environmental. Gut 17: 235–243 (1976).

3   Mayberry, J. F.; Rhodes, J.; Newcombe, R. G.: Familial prevalence of inflammatory bowel disease in relatives of patients with Crohn's disease. Br. med. J. i: 84 (1980).

4   Weterman, I. T.; Peña, A. S.: Familial incidence of Crohn's disease in the Netherlands and a review of the literature. Gastroenterology 86: 449–452 (1984).

5   Miller, D. S.; Keighley, A. C.; Langman, M. J. S.: Changing patterns in epidemiology of Crohn's disease. Lancet ii: 691–693 (1974).

6   Smith, I. S.; Young, S.; Gillespie. G.; O'Connor, J.; Bell, J. R.: Epidemiological aspects of Crohn's disease in Clydesdale 1961–1970. Gut 16: 62–67 (1975).

7   Mayberry, J. F.; Rhodes, J.; Hughes, L. E.: Incidence of Crohn's disease in Cardiff between 1934 and 1977. Gut 20: 602–608 (1979).

8   Devlin, H. B.; Datta, D.; Dellipiani, A. W.: The incidence and prevalence of inflammatory bowel disease in North Tees Health District. Wld J. Surg. 4: 183–193 (1980).

9   Mayberry, J. F.; Dew, M. J.; Morris, J. S.; Powell, D. B.: An audit of Crohn's disease in a defined population. J. R. Coll, Physns 17: 196–198 (1983).

10 Lee, F. I.; Costello, F. T.: Crohn's disease in Blackpool 1968–1980. Gut 26: 247–248 (1985).

11 Lockhart-Mummery, H. E.; Morson, B. C.: Crohn's disease (regional enteritis) of the large intestine and its distinction from ulcerative colitis. Gut 1: 87–105 (1960).

12 Lockhart-Mummery, H. E.; Morson, B. C.: Crohn's disease of the large intestine. Gut 5: 493–509 (1964).

13 Harries, A. D.; Baird, A.; Rhodes, J.; Mayberry, J. F.: Has the rising incidence of Crohn's disease reached a plateau? Br. med. J. i: 235 (1982).

14 Kyle, J.; Stark, G.: Fall in the incidence of Crohn's disease. Gut 21: 340–343 (1980).

15 Binder, V.; Both, H.; Hanson, P. K.; Hendriksen, C.; Kreiner, S.; Torp-Pendersen, K.: Incidence and prevalence of ulcerative colitis and Crohn's disease in the County of Copenhagen. Gastroenterology 83: 563–568 (1982).
16 Nunes, G. C.; Ahlquist, R. E.: Increasing incidence of Crohn's disease. Am. J. Surg. 145: 578–581 (1983).
17 Brahme, F.; Lindstrom, C.; Wenckert. A.: Crohn's disease in a defined population. Gastroenterology 69: 342–351 (1975).
18 Sedlack, R. E.; Whishant, J.; Elveback, L. R.; Kurland, L. T.: Incidence of Crohn's disease in Olmsted County, Minnesota 1935–1975. Am. J. Epidem. 112: 759–763 (1980).
19 Mayberry J. F.: Some aetiological factors in the epidemiology of Crohn's disease. Hepato-gastroenterol. 29: 167–168 (1982).
20 Mayberry, J. F.; Rhodes, J.: Epidemiological aspects of Crohn's disease: a review of the literature. Gut 25: 886–889 (1984).
21 Langman, M. J. S.: Inflammatory bowel disease. Incidence, epidemiology and genetics, in Bouchier, Allan, Hodgson, Keighley, Gastroenterology, p. 885 (Baillière Tindall, London 1984).

Frank I. Lee, MB, FRCP, Department of Gastroenterology, Victoria Hospital, Blackpool, Lancashire FY3 8NR (UK)

Front. gastrointest. Res., vol. 11, pp. 114–117 (Karger, Basel 1986)

The Changing Incidence of Crohn's Disease in Wales and the Role of Heredity in Its Aetiology

John Francis Mayberry[a], *John Rhodes*[b]

[a] Queens Medical Centre, University Hospital of Nottingham, UK;
[b] University Hospital of Wales, Cardiff, UK

In 1837, the Glamorgan and Monmouthshire Infirmary and Dispensary was opened and from that date records of patient admissions were kept. In 1926, Dr. *Robert Enoch* introduced a detailed diagnostic index which continues to the present [1]. His comments were prophetic when he wrote 'with time its value will increase'. It is because of the foresight of such physicians that we have been able to conduct a number of studies in the Cardiff area.

Studies of Incidence in Cardiff [2, 3]

The City of Cardiff is particularly suited for long-term retrospective studies. It has a relatively stable population and the medical records system with a diagnostic index has been carefully kept since 1926. The first study in Cardiff [2] was undertaken to see whether there had been an increase in incidence and if so what part of this could be attributed to an increase in the diagnosis of Crohn's colitis.

Between 1934 and 1977, 232 Cardiff residents were diagnosed as having Crohn's disease. The annual incidence rose from $0.18/10^5$/year during the period 1931–1935 to $4.83/10^5$/year during 1971–1975.

The rise in incidence cannot be attributed to: (1) better diagnostic facilities, as throughout this period there was an increase in the number of cases first diagnosed at surgery; (2) the diagnosis of milder cases, as mortality from Crohn's disease has remained constant throughout this time [4]; (3) confusion with ulcerative colitis – the incidence of ulcerative colitis has not changed [5] while that of Crohn's colitis has increased in parallel with that of ileocaecal disease, or (4) better retrieval and indexing of more recent cases – during the same period the incidence of achalasia [6] has not shown a similar rise in incidence (fig. 1).

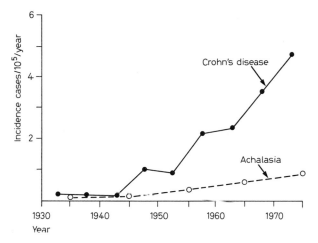

Fig. 1. The incidence of achalasia and Crohn's disease in Cardiff between 1930 and 1975.

Since 1975, the incidence of Crohn's disease has remained fairly stable at 4.9 cases/10^5/year [3].

Studies of Prevalence in Wales [7]

The prevalence of Crohn's disease in Cardiff is high at 56/10^5 population but it is typical of an urban community in the south-east of Wales. During the decade 1967–1976 about 1,100 patients from Wales were admitted to hospital with Crohn's disease. The majority of the cases came from the south-eastern counties of Glamorgan and Gwent (fig. 2).

The prevalence in urban communities was 47.6/10^5 compared with 34/10^5 in rural areas. Although this difference is significant and has been described in several studies it cannot be readily explained especially in an age when so many people commute regularly from homes in the country to work in industrial centres.

Studies in Rural Communities [8]

Ogwr is a small rural area 30 miles to the west of Cardiff. It has a fairly stable population of about 130,000 and is served by its own hospital. Between 1961 and 1980 79 patients were diagnosed as having Crohn's

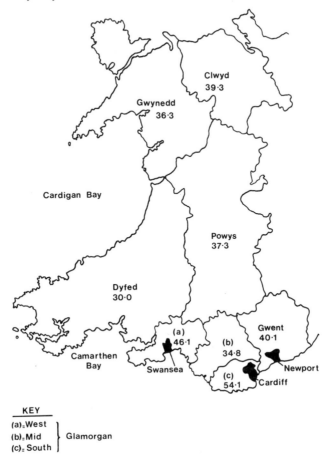

Fig. 2. The period prevalence of Crohn's disease in Welsh counties for the decade 1967–1976. Reproduced with permission from the Postgraduate Medical Journal.

disease and the incidence rose from $1.97/10^5$/year to $4.34/10^5$/year. This change parallels that seen in Cardiff and the increase in incidence of Crohn's disease appears to have occurred in both urban and rural communities and is independent of very sophisticated diagnostic techniques.

Family Studies of Crohn's Disease [9, 10]

Ninety five percent of patients resident in Cardiff were interviewed about the occurrence of inflammatory bowel disease in first-degree relatives. The prevalence in relatives is 13 times greater than in non-relatives and 30 times greater in siblings. These figures suggest that heredity plays a role in the aetiology of Crohn's disease, but not in a simple Mendelian fashion and it is likely that an external factor such as infection or diet plays a role.

Further evidence for some inherited element in the aetiology of Crohn's disease comes from a study of atopic disease [10]. Two hundred patients and controls were investigated and 36.5% of patients with Crohn's disease had a positive family history of atopic disease compared with only 10% of controls. However, patients had no greater frequency of asthma, hay fever or allergic rhinitis than controls.

Perhaps the patient with Crohn's disease is particularly susceptible to some environmental factor which has become more widespread in the 20th century and we can only echo the thoughts of *Dalzeil* [11] when he wrote: 'I trust cre long further consideration will clear up the difficulty.'

References

1   Mayberry, J. F.: The history of a hospital and its diagnostic index. Publ. Hlth. *93:* 311–316 (1976).
2   Mayberry, J. F.; Rhodes, J.; Hughes, L. E.: Incidence of Crohn's disease in Cardiff between 1934 and 1977. Gut *20:* 602–608 (1979).
3   Harries, A. D.; Baird, A.; Rhodes, J.; Mayberry, J. F.: Has the rising incidence of Crohn's disease reached a plateau? Br. med. J. *284:* 235 (1982).
4   Mayberry, J. F.; Newcombe, R. G.; Rhodes, J.: Mortality in Crohn's disease. Q. Jl Med. *49:* 65–68 (1980).
5   Morris, T. J.; Rhodes, J.: Incidence of proctocolitis in the Cardiff Region, 1968–1977. Gut *21:* A923 (1980).
6   Mayberry, J. F.; Rhodes, J.: Achalasia in the City of Cardiff from 1926 to 1977. Digestion *20:* 248–252 (1980).
7   Mayberry, J. F.; Rhodes, J.; Newcombe, R. G.: Crohn's disease in Wales, 1967–1976; an epidemiological survey based on hospital admissions. Post-grad. med. J. *56:* 336–341 (1980).
8   Mayberry, J. F.; Dew, M. J; Morris, J. S.; Powell, D. B.: An audit of Crohn's disease in a defined population. J. R. Coll. Physns of Lond. *17:* 196–198 (1983).
9   Mayberry, J. F.; Rhodes, J.; Newcombe, R. G.: Familial prevalence of inflammatory bowel disease in relatives of patients with Crohn's disease. Br. med. J. *1:* 84 (1980).
10 Pugh, S. M.; Rhodes, J.; Mayberry, J. F.; Roberts, D. L.; Heatley, R. V.; Newcombe, R. G.: Atopic disease in ulcerative colitis and Crohn's disease. Clin. Allergy *9:* 221–223 (1979).
11 Dalzeil, T. K.: Chronic interstitial enteritis. Br. med. J. *ii:* 1068–1070 (1913).

John Francis Mayberry, MD, MRCP, Queens Medical Centre, University Hospital of Nottingham, Nottingham NG7 2UH (UK)

Ethnic, Religious and Occupational Groups

Front. gastrointest. Res., vol. 11, pp. 118–134 (Karger, Basel 1986)

Chronic Inflammatory Bowel Disease in Immigrants in the United Kingdom

J. A. Walker-Smith[a], *G. F. A. Benfield*[b], *R. D. Montgomery*[b],
P. Asquith[b], *J. M. Findlay*[c], *S. D. Jayaratne*[c], *S. K. F. Chong*[a]

[a] St. Bartholomew's Hospital, London; [b] East Birmingham Hospital, and
[c] Bradford Royal Infirmary, UK

Introduction

There have been many large surveys of chronic inflammatory bowel disease based on the indigenous populations of Western countries [1–9]. However, there are relatively few studies originating elsewhere. Probably for this reason, ulcerative colitis and Crohn's disease have been regarded as uncommon or rare in tropical climates.

Nevertheless, over the last two decades several papers have appeared from India and Sri Lanka documenting a series of patients with ulcerative colitis [10–16], giving credence to the view that the disease is not so uncommon as was once thought in these populations. In contrast, reports of ulcerative colitis and Crohn's disease from the African continent remain sporadic [17] and it is thought to have remained uncommon in urban areas of Africa [18] and also in the USA where large indigenous black populations live [5]. Similarly, in the West Indies (Trinidad and Tobago) only one survey has appeared describing Indians and Negroes with inflammatory bowel disease [19]. Given the size of the Asian and African populations studied, the numbers described are not large and there is an absence of epidemiological data, so it has been impossible to draw conclusions regarding incidence and prevalence of chronic inflammatory bowel disease in these countries.

In Great Britain there are well-established communities of Indians, Pakistanis and West Indians (of African stock), but despite this, reports of chronic inflammatory bowel disease have been confined to two studies with small numbers [20, 21].

In this chapter the results of three different studies are reported. There are two studies of adult patients from Birmingham and Bradford and one study of child patients from London.

Chronic Inflammatory Bowel Disease in Immigrants in Birmingham

G. F. A. Benfield, R. D. Montgomery, P. Asquith
East Birmingham Hospital, Birmingham, UK

This summarizes a survey in the Birmingham area involving all immigrants who presented to the gastroenterology unit at the East Birmingham Hospital with either ulcerative colitis or Crohn's disease over a 15-year period. Fifty patients (30 males and 20 females: 22 Indians, 22 Pakistanis, 6 West Indians) were diagnosed as having either ulcerative colitis (44) or Crohn's disease (6) based on accepted clinical, histological and radiological criteria. This followed extensive blood and serological investigation for parasites and other bowel pathogens, namely *Salmonella* and *Shigella* species, *Mycobacterium tuberculosis*, *Yersinia enterocolitica* and *Campylobacter jejuni*.

Results

Age at Presentation

It was found that female patients presented significantly earlier than males (29.1 ± 2.5 vs. 38.9 ± 2.1 years, mean $\pm$ SEM) ($p < 0.01$) and this correlated with an earlier age of immigration to Great Britain rather than the female 'population' distribution as a whole (18.6 ± 1.8 vs. 26.8 ± 2.8 $p < 0.05$). Furthermore, the average time spent in this country before the onset of symptoms was the same in both sexes (9.6 ± 1.7 in females vs. 12.5 ± 1.6 in males, $p < 0.2$). Nine of our patients were second-generation immigrants and all had developed symptoms before the age of 20, a finding which was not wholly explained by the age distribution of the second generation population [22]. Again the mean age at onset of symptoms (10.9 ± 1.8) was identical to the latent period experienced by the first-generation immigrants (11.0 ± 1.7). This suggests that both environmental and racial influences may be involved in the generation of chronic inflammatory bowel disease in such populations. It is interesting that only two of the patients had developed symptoms prior to entering Great Britain.

Delay before Hospital Admission

There was a wide range of period of symptoms before patients attended hospital with a mean of 15 months (range 1 week to 12 years). One-quarter of the patients presented with symptoms lasting less than a

Table I. Extent of disease in patients with ulcerative colitis in Birmingham

	Rectum/recto-sigmoid	Distal/total colon
Pakistani	9	10
Indian	3	16
West Indian	1	5

month but 20%, mainly males, suffered symptoms for over 12 months before attending hospital. There are probably several reasons for this but in view of the prevalence of infective diarrhoea in Asians it is possible that many patients were simply treated with repeated courses of antibiotics and anti-diarrhoeals thus delaying the eventual correct diagnosis.

Blood Results

A particularly interesting phenomenon was the number of patients (17), all with ulcerative colitis, who presented with an eosinophilia. Extensive investigations failed to establish a parasitic aetiology, nor were there any atopic or other systemic disorders commonly associated with raised circulating eosinophil levels. There was no obvious explanation for this finding and it may represent a peculiar racial response to chronic inflammatory bowel disease, perhaps associated with some hypersensitivity or allergic phenomena occurring in the inflamed bowel. There have been many suggestions of hypersensitivity reactions to foreign proteins such as those derived from milk [23–25], and this may be a secondary phenomenon precipitated by the passage of many antigens across the inflamed mucosa. Certainly, the diet of such ethnic groups changes markedly on immigration and this may play some, as yet unidentified, role either in the aetiology of chronic inflammatory bowel disease or in the subsequent immunological response to established disease.

Site of Disease

The extent of large bowel involvement in the 44 patients with ulcerative colitis was studied and the patients were placed in one of three groups, either total colitis, left-sided colitis (where involvement was less than total but extended beyond the sigmoid colon) and either rectal or recto-sigmoidal involvement. The overall distribution was fairly even, but Indians had significantly more extensive disease than Pakistanis, most of whom had disease confined to the rectum or recto-sigmoid (table I). In contrast, all but one Indian patient with left-sided colitis had colonic involvement extending proximally to the splenic flexure. Studies from India suggest that distal disease is more common [10, 11, 15, 16], so there is a considerable discrepancy between the extent of disease within the indigenous population and those who have emigrated. Unfortunately, no figures are available from within Pakistan and in the only study from the West Indies [19], nearly half the patients had a total colitis with only 1 patient having disease confined to the rectum. However, the authors do not elaborate on the extent of the distal colitis.

Our 6 patients with Crohn's disease demonstrated a widely scattered degree of large and small bowel involvement; 1 had ileo-caecal involvement, 2 distal procto-colitis, 2 both large and small bowel involvement, and 1 had segmental small bowel disease.

Follow-Up

The mean period of follow-up of patients with ulcerative colitis was 2.5 years (range 3 months to 8.5 years) with 40% of patients defaulting. One of the problems of dealing with an immigrant population is that it is extremely mobile with many returning home to the Indian subcontinent either permanently or for long periods, often lasting several months. In contrast, although few in number, none of our patients with Crohn's disease defaulted and were followed up for a mean period of nearly 5 years (range 1–12 years), perhaps because of the different nature of the disease and its symptomatology.

Pregnancy

Sixteen females were of childbearing age at the time of symptoms. During the course of follow-up, 9 (56%) became pregnant, 2 of them twice, and 2 of them on three occasions. The period of follow-up of such patients is short (3.1 ± 2 years) compared to an earlier study in whites which recorded a pregnancy rate of only 31% over a 12-year period, and this would suggest that pregnancy in our ethnic groups is not unduly influenced by chronic inflammatory bowel disease. Again this might suggest cultural influences, particularly in Asians where greater store is placed on large families.

Course of Disease and Treatment

Contrary to a large study within the indigenous population of Great Britain [3], we found that considerably more of our immigrants with ulcerative colitis (57%) experienced a single attack of symptoms followed by remission, 32% had a relapsing/remitting course and only 11% suffered a chronic, continuous illness, with poorly controlled symptoms. This seems to indicate a milder disease perhaps due to the widespread use of oral sulphasalazine and oral and topical corticosteroids, which were

Table II. Complications of ulcerative colitis and Crohn's disease in Birmingham (31 patients)

Local	
Acute toxic dilatation	5
Fistula	3 (Crohn's 2)
Colonic stricture	1 (Crohn's)
Perianal abscess	1 (crohn's)
Rectal prolapse	1
Systemic	
Anaemia (< 10 g/dl)	16 (Crohn's 1)
Arthropathy	5
Cutaneous disorders	6 (Crohn's 1)
Oral ulcers	4
Hepatitis	2
Haematological	2
Sulphasalazine sensitivity	3
Ophthalmological	1

perhaps not quite so evident in the earlier surveys. Use was also made of low residue milk-free or low-milk diets. Alternatively, the disease might be milder in Asians and this has been suggested by some of the Indian studies [11, 16], but not others [10, 15]. In contrast, *Bartholomew and Butler* [19] regarded the disease in Trinidad as more severe with a higher incidence of complications, and this was reflected in our own experience of our 6 West Indian patients with ulcerative colitis. Four suffered severe, relapsing disease, and 2 patients developed a toxic megacolon, one possibly due to Salazopyrin® sensitivity. In all, 3 patients developed a sensitivity to Salazopyrin, a reaction not clinically demonstrated in our Asian patients. One patient had, at an early age, been operated on for repeated gastrointestinal bleeding and was found to have benign lymphoid hyperplasia. One patient developed a persistent neutropenia. All patients have as a result had repeated hospital admissions for either their bowel disease or complications; again this experience is at variance to that of the Asians.

Complications and Mortality

Despite the relatively mild disease overall of our patients, the incidence of complications was high with 31 patients (62%) affected (table II), accentuated by the relatively short period of follow-up. These figures contrast with those of earlier surveys [27–29] where lower numbers of patients developed complications, although proportionately more suffered local, colonic lesions. This might reflect a longer period of follow-up compared to that in our immigrants. The complications, however, although frequent tended to be mild and consisted mainly of mild to moderate degrees of anaemia, arthritis and oral ulceration. In all, 17 patients experienced one complication, 10 had two, but in 4 cases complications were multiple, with 1 patient (West Indian) suffering a combination of acute toxic dilatation, leucoerythroblastic anaemia, sulphasalazine sensitivity and arthritis. Local complications of the bowel were few, the main ones being an acute toxic dilatation in 5 patients (3 West Indian).

There were 4 deaths, 2 from sepsis following a panprocto-colectomy for fulminant disease, a third patient from bleeding varices secondary to chronic active hepatitis and a fourth patient from a coexistant IgG myeloma.

Cultural Aspects

Other less-tangible problems arose during the management of our patients. Apart from the problems of follow-up, those who did attend the clinic demonstrated variable problems with communication. Nearly half of the female Asians could not speak English and required an accompanying interpreter, the provision of which was not always guaranteed. Most of the male Asians could speak English and certainly all West Indians were fluent. The discrepancy reflects cultural mores as females are discouraged from outside employment and contact with English-speaking groups, thus maintaining a perpetual language problem. Furthermore, the concept of chronic illness was not readily accepted by many patients and this led to problems with out-patient management together with the use by the patients of alternative therapies such as those provided by 'hakims'. This often resulted in difficulty in impressing on the patients the nature of the disease and the necessity for prophylactic therapy and long-term follow-up, problems which might be overcome with the use of a Health Visitor attached to the clinic in a similar fashion to that of tuberculosis clinics, where poor compliance can be reversed with home visits.

Conclusions

The presentation and clinical course of chronic inflammatory bowel disease in the Asian and West Indian communities of Birmingham was studied over a 15-year period. Disease remains uncommon but relatively severe in those patients of African extraction but occurs more frequently, mildly and with a high incidence of complications in Asians. The onset of symptoms occurs at an age reflecting the age at immigration and appears to present earlier in second generation immigrants. A large number of patients presented with a blood eosinophilia.

Most patients from Pakistan have disease confined to the distal large bowel whereas Indian patients suffer more extensive disease although this was not reflected by the clinical activity. Forty percent of patients with ulcerative colitis defaulted from follow-up, a feature thought likely to reflect cultural and ethnic influences. It was the overall impression that chronic inflammatory bowel disease in immigrants in Birmingham behaves differently to that in white populations.

Chronic Inflammatory Bowel Disease in the Asian Community in Bradford

J. M. Findlay, S. D. Jayaratne
Bradford Royal Infirmary, Bradford, UK

The Bradford District Hospitals serve a population of some 347,000 people of whom 42,300 are of immigrant origin, mainly of Asian extraction from Pakistan, India, Bangladesh, South Africa, Kenya and Uganda.

A retrospective study was carried out examining the pattern and prevalence of ulcerative colitis and Crohn's disease within the immigrant population between the years 1968 and 1983. The information described below was obtained from a review of Hospital Activity Analysis in the two District General Hospitals. Due allowance has been made reaching our final numbers for patients who have, in fact, attended both hospitals.

All the case-notes classified under chronic inflammatory bowel disease in the two Hospitals were retrieved from the beginning of 1968 to the end of 1983. They included all admissions and clinic patients. From these patients originating from the Indian subcontinent were selected. Before these patients were included in the study strict diagnostic criteria for both Crohn's disease and ulcerative colitis were applied. Characteristic sigmoidoscopic or colonoscopic and radiological appearances, together with unequivocal histology were necessary before any patient could be included. All those patients with bowel pathogens; Campylobacter, Salmonella, Shigella, Amoebi and acid-fast bacilli were excluded.

A postal questionnaire was sent to all patients for further information, but this data has not been included in view of the very poor response rate.

Table III. Clinical features of 37 Asian patients with chronic inflammatory bowel disease in Bradford

Symptoms	Number of cases	
	ulcerative colitis	Crohn's disease
Diarrhoea	25	4
Blood and mucus	25	3
Abdominal pain	15	6
Weight loss	14	5
Anorexia/vomiting	8	0
Abdominal tenderness	6	4
Abdominal mass or thickened bowel	1	4

A total of 37 immigrant patients was retrieved for the study. Of these 37 patients, 25 were males and 12 females. Twenty-nine of the patients had ulcerative colitis and 8 had Crohn's disease. Of the patients with ulcerative colitis there were 19 males and 10 females. Of the patients with Crohn's disease there were 6 males and 2 females.

Twenty-two of the patients were Pakistani Muslims and of these, 17 had ulcerative colitis and 5 Crohn's disease. Twelve of the 15 patients from India had ulcerative colitis and 3 had Crohn's disease. The majority appeared to be immigrant textile workers although the occupational history was not complete in all. None of the patients had symptoms suggestive of a bowel disorder before coming to the United Kingdom. There was no family history of similar disorders and none of the patients gave a history of significant illness including tuberculosis.

The prevalence of ulcerative colitis and Crohn's disease was some 78 per 100,000 of the immigrant population. The figure for ulcerative colitis was 59 per 100,000 of the population, and 15 per 100,000 of population with Crohn's disease.

Clinical Features

The presenting clinical features are shown in table III. It can be seen that the major clinical manifestations are diarrhoea and the presence of blood in the stools. Abdominal pain was a feature of all Crohn's disease patients. None had fever at presentation. Associated systemic problems were few. One patient had an arthritis of both knee joints and 2 had backache with radiological evidence of a sacro-ileitis.

Table IV. Laboratory findings in Bradford

Investigations	Ulcerative colitis		Crohn's disease	
	mean	range	mean	range
Hb, g/dl	8.75	15.5–3.8	12.9	16.8–9.2
ESR, mm/h	21.96	74–1	33.12	88–1
WCC × 10⁹/l	8.1	17.5–2.7	10.4	15.6–6.0
T proteins, g/l	72.2	85–60	66.1	75–54
Platelets × 10⁹/l	501	600–225	496	642–283
Albumin, g/l	39.6	48–24	37.8	53–17

Laboratory Investigations

The laboratory investigations are presented in table IV. The haemoglobin was below 12 g in 18 patients (48%). Two patients with Crohn's disease and 2 patients with ulcerative colitis had haemoglobins below 6 g at presentation. The ESR was significantly raised, i.e. over 50 mm/h, in 2 patients only. Eight patients were in the range between 30 and 50 mm/h. The serum albumin was below the normal range in 6 patients with marked reduction to 1.7 g/l in 1 patient. The only other common laboratory abnormality was the low serum iron of ferritin level in 11 patients. The white cell count was over $12 \times 10^9/l$ in only 1 patient at presentation, and no patient had significant liver enzyme changes.

The Extent and Distribution of Bowel Involvement

Ulcerative Colitis (fig. 1). Nine patients out of the series of 29 patients with ulcerative colitis presented with total confluent colitis. Figure 1 indicates the distribution of the disease in the colon of patients with ulcerative colitis. It can be seen that the disease tended to become less frequent, as one might expect, as observation was made from the rectum proximally.

Crohn's Disease (fig. 2). One patient had total confluent colitis and here the disease can be seen to be somewhat more frequent the more proximal one moved around the colon with a maximum frequency being found in the ileo-caecal area.

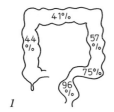 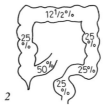

Fig. 1. Distribution expressed as a percentage in 29 patients treated for ulcerative colitis.

Fig. 2. Distribution expressed as a percentage in 8 patients treated for Crohn's disease.

Outcome of Disease

The problems of following up the Asian patients were considerable, as they tended to be a fairly ambulant population. Efforts at checking patients' whereabouts were much complicated by the patients' mobility within the Bradford district alone; their tendency to move out of the Bradford district to other parts of the country, the reluctance on the part of many patients to attent the follow-up clinic, and, finally, there were problems of recalling patients in view of the similarity of their names.

The need for surgery in the patients with ulcerative colitis and Crohn's disease was considerable. No less than 24% of our patients with ulcerative colitis ended up with surgery; 4 undergoing pan-proctocolectomies, 2 with ileo-rectal anastomoses and 1 went on to subsequent removal of the rectum. Of the patients with Crohn's disease, four patients underwent right hemicolectomy.

Discussion

The male to female ratio characteristic of the Bradford series is a reflection of the male to female ratio of the immigrant community as a whole. In the early 1960s the Asian population was almost entirely male.

Towards the end of the 1970s families and next of kin started coming into the country in increasing numbers, but there was still a significant male to female preponderance within the community.

This retrospective study suggests that chronic inflammatory bowel disease amongst the immigrant Asian community may not be as uncommon as perhaps previously expected. This contrasts with the relatively few epidemiological studies from India, Pakistan and South East Asia [10–12, 14, 16, 30–32], which show a low incidence of chronic inflammatory bowel disease in comparison with Western societies. There are certain difficulties in interpreting the epidemiological data from developing countries due to several factors; firstly, the difference in levels of ascertainment of disease are considerable between developed and developing countries due to patient attitude, access to medical care and availability of diagnosatic facilities. Secondly, there are variations in diagnostic practices in different countries where amoebic and bacillary dysentery are common compared with those where they are not [33].

There may be differences in population structure. Non-industrial countries have a greater proportion of younger age groups than industrial countries. Although we could not establish a temporal relationship between the duration of stay in the United Kingdom in our patients and the onset of disease, it is particularly relevant that none of the patients presented with the disease on arrival in this country. The presentation of the disease and the laboratory findings would appear to be exactly what one would expect in the indigenous population with chronic inflammatory bowel disease. The number of patients with total colonic involvement with ulcerative colitis is probably higher than seen in the indigenous Bradford community, and the striking need for surgery would suggest that when the disease does present, it seems to persue a more aggressive course than would be typical of that found in the indigenous community.

The increased prevalence of the disease, and the severity of the pattern of disease in the immigrant population compared with the population on the Asian sub-continent [34–37], is difficult to explain. It may well be the stress of emigration itself, or the social pressure put on the patients when they arrive in this country. Others have suggested that it may be the change in moving from a rural to an industrial environment.

Whilst this study has confined itself to chronic inflammatory bowel disease in the Asian community in Bradford, and only considered ulcerative colitis and Crohn's disease, it is extremely relevant to remember that almost twice the number of patients described in this series suffering from tuberculosis of the gastrointestinal tract have been seen over a similar period [38].

Chronic Inflammatory Bowel Disease in Children from the Asian Immigrant Community in London

S. K. F. Chong, and J. A. Walker-Smith

St. Bartholomew's Hospital, London, UK

In the London area over the last 8 years from July 1975 to October 1983, 124 children have been reviewed in the Paediatric Inflammatory Bowel Disease Clinic at St. Bartholomew's Hospital. There were altogether 17 Asian children diagnosed as chronic inflammatory bowel disease based on a combination of clinical, radiological, endoscopic and histological criteria [39].

Five Asian children had Crohn's disease (4 male, 1 female) whilst 10 had ulcerative colitis (5 male, 5 female). Two children (1 male, 1 female) had the diagnosis of intestinal Behçet's disease made following histopathological examination of their resected colons [40].

The 10 Asian children with ulcerative colitis comprised 35.7% of the total number of children in the study period. The 5 children with Crohn's disease made up to 6.7% of the total number seen (fig. 3).

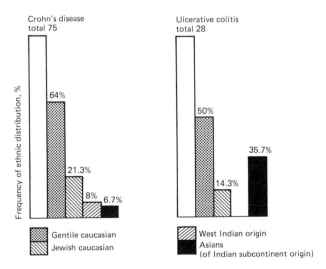

Fig. 3. Racial and ethnic distribution of children with chronic inflammatory bowel disease at St. Bartholomew's Hospital, London.

Table V. Crohn's disease in London Asian children

Name	Age	Sex	Origins	Place of birth
F. D.	5	M	Hyderabad, Andhra Pradesh	UK
A. M.	13	F	Jabalpur, Madya Pradesh	UK
A. S.	16	M	Punjab	UK
R. K.	4	M	Silat, Bangladesh	UK
A. K.	12	M	Karachi, Pakistan	Karachi

Table VI. Dietary pattern in Crohn's disease in London Asian children

Name	Age	Sex	Diet	Family history	Travel prior to illness
F. D.	5	M	traditional and westernised	–	never been to India
A. M.	13	F	traditional and westernised	–	never been to India
A. S.	16	M	traditional	–	been to India
R. K.	4	M	traditional and westernised	–	never been to India
A. K.	12	M	traditionai	–	lives in Abu Dhabi

The ages of the 5 children with Crohn's disease ranged from 4 to 16 years. Although their origins were from the northern and central Indian subcontinent, all the children, except one, were born in the United Kingdom (table V).

Only two of the children had ever been to India. Three of the children were on a traditional and westernised diet, and two were taking a traditional diet (table VI). None of the children had a family history of chronic inflammatory bowel disease.

The ages of the 10 children with ulcerative colitis ranged from 3 to 14 years. Two were born in the Indian subcontinent in Boroda and Silat (table VII). All the others were born in the United Kingdom. In 2 cases, 1 of the parents had come from Uganda originally. The others originated from the North Indian subcontinent. Five of the 10 children had been to India on some occasion. There was a variable dietary pattern, i.e. traditional or westernised (table VIII). Only 1 child with ulcerative colitis had a family history, namely her father.

Table VII. Ulcerative colitis in London Asian children

Name	Age	Sex	Origins	Place of Birth
J. V.	12	F	Ludhiana, Punjab	UK
H. M.	11	F	Boroda, Gujerat	Boroda
T. J.	9	F	Uganda & Gujerat	UK
S. K.	14	M	Marachi, Pakistan	UK
S. G.	12	F	Hoshiarpur Punjab	UK
S. B.	5	M	Silat, Bangladesh	Silat
S. P.	11	F	Gujerat & Uganda	UK
G. B.	6	M	Karachi, Pakistan	UK
A. H.	3	M	India	UK
K. K.	14	M	Maharashtra	UK

Table VIII. Dietary pattern in ulcerative colitis in Asian children

Name	Age	Sex	Diet	Family history	Travel prior to illness
J. V.	12	F	traditional and westernised	–	been to Punjab 2 years ago
H. M.	11	F	traditional	father (UC)	been to India 6 months before
T. J.	9	F	traditional and westernised	–	never been to India
S. K.	14	M	traditional and westernised	–	never been to India
S. G.	12	F	traditional (vegetarian)	–	been to India twice, but well
S. B.	5	M	traditional	–	at age 3.5 years had dysentry in Bangladesh
S. P.	11	F	traditional and westernised	–	never been to India
G. B.	6	M	traditional	–	been in Pakistan 3 years ago for 1 year
A. H.	3	M	traditional (vegetarian)	–	never been to India
K. K.	14	M	westernised	–	never been to India

Two children were dignosed as intestinal Behcet's disease based on histopathology of the resected colon, which showed virtually identical features of multiple deep flask-shaped ulcers in the presence of chronic inflammation, without any of the characteristic histological features of Crohn's disease. These 2 children were born of first cousin Pakistani parents. They subsequently improved following subtotal colectomy and are presently well with intermittent diarrhoea [40].

This small series of children with chronic inflammatory bowel disease suggest that both ulcerative colitis and Crohn's disease occur not infrequently in Asian children of immigrant families in the United Kingdom, although there has been a scarcity of reports of this disease in children living in the Indian subcontinent.

Other Racial and Ethnic Groups

There are no West Indian children who had ulcerative colitis, although 6 had Crohn's disease [41]. A caseof Crohn's disease in a West Indian infant has previously been published from the unit [42]. Jewish children accounted for 21.3% of children with Crohn's disease and 14.3% of those with ulcerative colitis, a disproportionate percentage for their overall representation in the population.

References

1   Bockus, H. L.; Roth, J. L. A.; Buchman, E.; Kalser, M.; Staub, W. R.; Finkelstein, A.; Valdes-Dapna, A.: Life history of non-specific ulcerative colitis: relation of prognosis to anatomical and clinical varieties. Gastroenterologia, Basel 86: 549–581 (1956).

2   Banks, B. M.; Dorelitz, B. I.; Zetzel, L.: The course of non-specific ulcerative colitis: review of twenty years experience and late results. Gastroenterology 32: 983–1012 (1957).

3   Edwards, F. C.; Truelove, S. C.: The course and prognosis of ulcerative colitis. Gut 4: 299–315 (1964).

4   Evans, J. G.; Acheson, E. D.: An epidemiological study of ulcerative colitis and regional enteritis in the Oxford area. Gut 6: 311–325 (1965).

5   Monk, M.; Mendeloff, A. I.; Siegel, C. I.; Lilienfeld, A.: An epidemiological study of ulcerative colitis and regional enteritis among adults in Baltimore. I. Hospital incidence and prevalence, 1960 to 1963. Gastroenterology 53: 198–210 (1967).

6   Bonnevie, O.; Riis, P.; Anthonisen, P.: An epidemiological study of ulcerative colitis in Copenhagen County. Scand. J. Gastroent. 3: 432–438 (1968).

7   Fahrlander, H.; Baerlocher, C. H.: Clinical features and epidemiological data on Crohn's disease in the Basle area. Scand. J. Gastroent. 6: 657–672 (1971).

8   Brahme, F.; Lindstrom, C.; Wenckert, A.: Crohn's disease in a defined population. An epidemiological study of incidence, prevalence, mortality and secular trends in the city of Malmo, Sweden. Gastroenterology 69: 342–351 (1975).

9   Gilat, T.; Lilos, P.; Zemishlany, Z.; Ribak, J.; Benaroya, Y.: Ulcerative colitis in the Jewish population of Tel-Aviv-Yafo. III. Clinical course. Gastroenterology 70: 14–19 (1976).

10 Tandon, B. N.; Mathur, A. K.; Mohapatra, L. N.; Tandon, H. D.; Wit, K. L.: A study of the prevalence and clinical pattern of non-specific ulcerative colitis in Northern India. Gut 6: 448–453 (1965).

11 Chuttani, H. K.; Nigam, S. P.; Sama, S. K.; Dhanda, P. C.; Gupta, P. S.: Ulcerative colitis in the tropics. Br. med. J. ii: 204–207 (1974).

12 Chopra, R. N ; Ray, R. N.: Indian med. Gaz. *74:* 65 (1939).

13 Nagaratnam, N.; Sheriffdeen, A. H.; Chetiawardene, A, D.; Rajiyah, S.; Wijesundera, A.: Ulcerative colitis in Sri-Lanka Patients. Trop. Doct. *11:* 52–54 (1981).

14 Mayberry, J. F.: Crohn's disease in developing countries. Ital. J. Gastro. *12:* 324 326 (1980).

15 Pimparkar, B. D.: Ulcerative colitis in Bombay. J. Indian med. Ass. *61:* 217–222 (1973).

16 Maroo, M. K.; Nag, N. K.; Sortur, S. V.; Patil, R. S.: Ulcerative colitis in Southern Maharashtra. J. Indian med. Ass. *63:* 350–354 (1974).

17 Billinghurst, J. R.; Welchman, J. M.: Idiopathic ulcerative colitis in the African: a report of four cases. Br. med. J. *i:* 211–213 (1966).

18 Walker, A. R. P.; Segal, I.: Epidemiology of non-infective intestinal disease in various ethnic groups in South Africa. Israel J. med. Scis *15:* 309–313 (1979).

19 Bartholomew, C.; Butler, A.: Inflammatory bowel disease in the West Indies. Br. med. J. *ii:* 824–825 (1979).

20 O'Donoghue, D. P.; Clark, M. L.: Inflammatory bowel disease in West Indians. Br. med. J. *ii:* 796 (1976).

21 Das, S. K.; Montgomery, R. D.: Chronic inflammatory bowel disease in Asian immigrants. Practitioner *221:* 747–749 (1978).

22 Census 1981: County report, West Midlands Part I, p. 19 (HMSO, London, 1982).

23 Taylor, K. B; Truelove, S. C.: Circulating antibodies to milk proteins in ulcerative colitis. Br. med J *ii;* 924–929 (1961).

24 Wright, R.; Truelove, S. C.: A controlled therapeutic trial of various diets in ulcerative colitis. Br. med. J. *ii:* 138–141 (1965).

25 Wright, R.; Truelove, S. C.: Circulating and tissue eosiniphils in ulcerative colitis. Am. J. dig. Dis *11:* 831–846 (1966).

26 Dombal, F. T. de; Watts, J. M.; Watkinson, G.; Goligher, J. C.: Ulcerative colitis and pregnancy. Lancet *2:* 599–602 (1965).

27 Ricketts, W. E.; Palmer, W. L.: Complications of chronic non-specific ulcerative colitis. Gastroenterology *7:* 55–66 (1946).

28 Dennis, C.; Karlson, K. E.: Surgical measures as supplements to the management of idiopathic ulcerative colitis; cancer, cirrhosis and arthritis as frequent complications. Surgery *32:* 892–912 (1952).

29 Greenstein, A. J.; Janowitz, H. D.; Sachar, D. B.: The extra-intestinal complications of Crohn's disease and ulcerative colitis: a study of 700 patients. Medicine *55:* 401–412 (1976).

30 Japanese Research Committee for Crohn's disease in Japan. Gastroenterol. jap. *14:* 367 (1979).

31 Ti, T. K.: Inflammatory disease of bowel. A Malasian experience. Aust. N. Z. J. Surg. *49:* 428–431 (1979).

32 Yang, Y. C.; Wh, Y. B.: Seminar in inflammatory bowel disease. Chin. J. Gastro. *1:* 44–49 (1981).

33 Tedesco, F. J.; Hardin, R. D.; Harper, R. N.; Edwards, B. H.: Infectious colitis endoscopically simulating inflammatory bowel disease. A prospective evaluation. Gastrointest. Endosc. *29:* 195 (1983).

34 Venagopadan, S.; Radhakrishnan, S.; Rajachandrasekaran, R.: Crohn's disease, a study of 21 cases. S. Indian J. Surg. *1980:* 42.

35 Tariq, A. M.; Sarwar, J. Z.: Ulcerative colitis. A retrospective study. J. Pak. med. Ass. *30:* 141–145 (1980).

36 Gupta, R. S.; Chatterjee, A. K.; Roy, R.; Ghoush, B. N.: A review of the results of treatment in 44 cases of Crohn's disease. Ind. J. Surg. *24:* 797–805 (1962).

37 Pastricha, K. K.; Chuttani, P. N.; Vidyasagar: J. Ass. Physcns, India *1:* 19 (1958).
38 Wig, J. D.; Nair, P. M.; Srinath, B. S.; Saleem, M A.; Katariya, R. N.; Bhusnurmuth, S. R.; Talwar, B. L.: Stenotic lesions of the bowel. Ind. J. Surg. *41:* 322–330 (1979).
39 Chong, S. K. F.; Blackshaw, A. J.; Boyle, S.; Williams, C. B.; Walker-Smith, J. A.: Histological diagnosis of chronic inflammatory bowel disease in childhood. Gut *26:* 55–60 (1984).
40 Chong, S. K. F.; Sanderson, I. R.; Walker-Smith, J. A.: Food allergy and infantile colitis (letter). Arch. Dis. Childh. *59:* 690–691 (1984).
41 Chong, S. K. F.; Walker-Smith, J. A.: Chronic inflammatory bowel disease in the young. Compreh. Ther. *8:* 27–34 (1982).
42 Wallis, S. M.; Walker-Smith, J. A.: An unusual case of Crohn's disease in a West Indian Child. Acta paediat. scand. *65:* 749 (1976).

J. A. Walker-Smith, MD, Department of Child Health, St. Bartholomew's
Hospital, West Smithfield, London EC1A 7BE (UK)

Front. gastrointest. Res., vol. 11, pp. 135–140 (Karger, Basel 1986)

Inflammatory Bowel Disease in Jews

T. Gilat, A. Grossman, Z. Fireman, P. Rozen

Department of Gastroenterology, Ichilov Hospital and Sackler Faculty of Medicine, Tel-Aviv University, Tel-Aviv, Israel

Interest in the incidence of inflammatory bowel disease (IBD) in Jews arose from studies performed in the USA in the early 1960s. *Acheson* [1] and *Weiner and Lewis* [2] reported in 1960 a 3- to 4-times higher incidence of ulcerative colitis (UC) in Jews among hospitalized US Army veterans. *Acheson and Nefzger* [3] analyzed, in 1963, the incidence of ulcerative colitis in US Army personnel during 1944. They found a twofold higher incidence in Jews. These surveys were obviously not population studies. *Monk* et al. [4] studied the incidence of UC and Crohn's disease (CD) in hospitalized patients in a defined population in Baltimore. They found a 3- to 4-times higher incidence in Jews for both diseases. The authors themselves raised the question of hospitalization bias and diagnostic bias. A higher incidence of both UC and CD in Jews in the USA was also noted by other investigators mainly in series from major medical centers [5, 6].

Gilat et al. [7] reported in 1974 an incidence of UC in Jews in Tel-Aviv which was lower than that reported for the general population in several part of Europe and probably lower than in the white population in the USA.

The above studies served to focus scientific interest on the incidence of IBD in Jews. In population studies performed in several parts of the world, mainly in Europe, particular attention was directed to the incidence of both diseases in Jews. The results of these studies are summarized below.

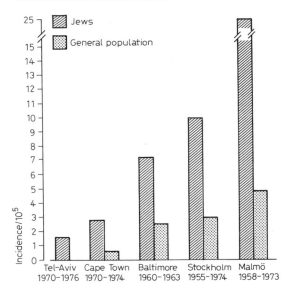

Fig. 1. Incidence (per 10⁵) of Crohn's disease in Jews and the general population in population studies in 5 geographic locations.

Incidence of IBD in Jews in Population Studies

Figure 1 shows the incidence of CD in Jews and in the general populations of Tel-Aviv [7], Cape Town [8], Baltimore [4], Stockholm [9] and Malmö [10]. The study in Baltimore is the only one to be based on hospitalized cases. Several facts stand out: (1) The incidence of CD in Jews in the various locations varies tremendously, the difference between Tel-Aviv and Malmö being almost 15-fold! (2) The increasing incidence in the Jews seems to parallel the rising incidence in the general population of the various areas Malmö > Stockholm > Baltimore > Capetown. (3) In all the above four cities, the incidence of CD in Jews is considerably higher than in the general population of the area.

Figure 2 shows similar data for UC in Tel-Aviv [4], Cape Town [8] and Baltimore [4]. Although fewer populations were studied the trend is quite similar to that found for CD.

For comparison, figure 3 shows the prevalence of a genetic (autosomal recessive) trait, primary adult lactase deficiency, in Jews of Tel-Aviv [11], New Haven, Connecticut [12] and Vancouver [13]. Unlike the findings in IBD the prevalence of this genetic trait in Jews in these three widely separated areas is almost identical.

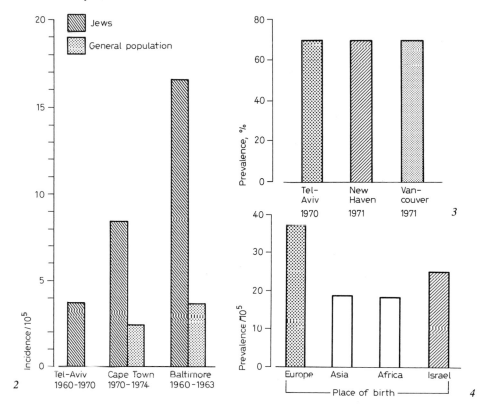

Fig. 2. Incidence (per 10^5) of ulcerative colitis in Jews and the general population in population studies in 3 geographic locations.

Fig. 3. Prevalence (%) of primary lactase deficiency in Jews in 3 geographic locations.

Fig. 4. Prevalence (per 10^5) of ulcerative colitis in the Jewish population of Israel by place of birth.

Figure 4 shows the prevalence of UC in Jews in Israel [7]. The prevalence is about 2 times higher in Jewish immigrants from Europe (a higher incidence area) than in immigrants from Africa and Asia (low incidence areas). The Jewish immigrants from Africa came mostly from northern Africa and those from Asia came mostly from Middle Eastern countries. The prevalence in Jews born in Israel was closer to that found in immigrants from the Middle East.

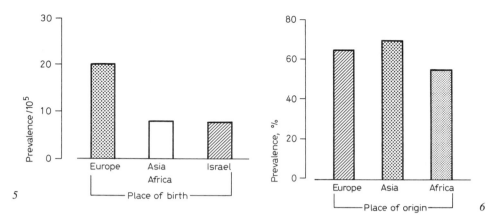

Fig. 5. Prevalence (per 10^5) of Crohn's disease in the Jewish population of Israel by place of birth.

Fig. 6. Prevalence (%) of primary lactase deficiency in the Jewish population of Israel by place of origin.

Figure 5 shows similar data for CD [14]. Again, the prevalence in Jews born in Europe was twice higher than in those born in Asia-Africa or Israel.

For comparison figure 6 shows the prevalence of primary adult lactase deficiency in the Jewish population of Israel [11]. The differences among the same 3 groups are minimal.

Discussion

When evaluating the data on the incidence of IBD in Jews in various parts of the world a difficulty arises. The number of Jews residing in some areas such as Malmö or Stockholm is not known with certainty and is relatively small. This is a source of inaccuracies. However, in other areas such as Baltimore, Capetown and Tel-Aviv, the numbers are relatively large and known with much greater certainty. Even if only these 3 areas were included in figure 1, the overall trend would not be altered.

The data in figures 1 and 2 strongly suggest the simultaneous effect of two factors. Environmental factors seem to predominate in view of the very marked differences in the incidence of IBD in Jews in the various geographic locations. The rising incidence in parallel with that in the general population of the various areas supports this interpretation. The fact that a genetic trait (lactase deficiency) does not show this variation but a rather marked uniformity also supports the predominance of environmental factors in the causation of IBD.

It is also clear, however, that in all these meticulously performed population studies the incidence of both UC and CD in Jews is higher than in the general population, supporting the earlier findings in the USA. This higher incidence in Jews may be caused by a genetic predisposition to IBD or by environmental factors (dietary, behavioral, familial) particular to Jews. Several considerations point towards the genetic hypothesis. The higher incidence in Jews was found in widely differing locations. Jews resided in these areas for different periods of time ranging from decades to centuries. Their integration and assimilation in the general population was not uniform or similar in the various areas. Thus, the denominator common to Jews in all these areas was their shared genetic background, rather than their environment. Present day scientific opinion holds that Jews share a common genetic pool [15, 16], as exemplified by studies of lactase deficiency (fig. 3).

The prevalence of lactase deficiency in the white population of the USA and Canada is mostly below 10%. Jews immigrated to these two countries 1–2 generations ago, mostly from Eastern Europe where they had lived for centuries. The prevalence of lactase deficiency in Eastern Europe is even lower than in the USA. Yet Jews have retained the prevalence of lactase deficiency of 60–70% found in their Mediterranean area of origin in Arabs, Southern Greeks and Italians [17].

Thus, the high and variable incidence of IBD in Jews the world over can best be explained by the interaction of 2 sets of factors: an increased predisposition to the disease(s), possibly genetic, and a more marked effect of environmental factor(s).

The study of IBD in Jews in Israel also demonstrates the effect of environmental factors (a genetic predisposition cannot be demonstrated in the absence of a control population). The disease(s) is more frequent in migrants from high incidence areas than in those from low incidence areas. The new generation born in Israel shows the lower incidence seen in migrants from Middle Eastern countries.

When the cause of a disease is unknown and unidentified environmental factors are suspected, the classical approach is to study migrant populations. Jews offer a unique group from this point of view having migrated over the centuries to various parts of the world. The study of the epidemiology of UC and CD in Jews offers strong support to the view that environmental factors are paramount in the causation of IBD. It also suggests the coexistence of genetic factors.

References

1   Acheson, E. D.: The distribution of ulcerative colitis and regional enteritis in United States veterans with particular reference to the Jewish religion. Gut *1:* 291–293 (1960).

2   Weiner, H. A.; Lewis, C. M.: Some notes on the epidemiology of nonspecific ulcerative colitis, an apparent increase in incidence in Jews. Am. J. dig. Dis. *5:* 406–418 (1960).

3   Acheson, E. D.; Nefzger, M. D.: Ulcerative colitis in the United States Army in 1944. Epidemiology: comparisons between patients and controls. Gastroenterology *44:* 7–19 (1963).

4   Monk, M.; Mendeloff, A. I.; Siegel, C. I.; Lilienfeld, A.: An epidemiological study of ulcerative colitis and regional enteritis among adults in Baltimore. I. Hospital incidence and prevalence, 1960–1963. Gastroenterology *53:* 198–210 (1967).

5   Korelitz, B. I.: Observation on the familial and ethnic aspects of Crohn's disease and ulcerative colitis in New York city; in Programme and Abstracts, Int. Workshop Epidemiology and Genetics of Inflammatory Bowel Disease, Liverpool 1983, Glaxo Symp., pp. 25–28.

6   Rogers, B. H. G.; Clark, L. M.; Kirsner, J. B.: The epidemiologic and demographic characteristics of inflammatory bowel disease. An analysis of a computerized file of 1400 patients. J. chron. Dis. *24:* 743–773 (1971).

7   Gilat, T.; Ribak, J.; Benaroya, Y.; Zemishlany, Z.; Weissman, I.: Ulcerative colitis in the Jewish population of Tel-Aviv Jafo. I. Epidemiology. Gastroenterology *66:* 335–342 (1974).

8   Novis, B. H.; Marks, I. N.; Bank, S.; Louw, H. J.: Incidence of Crohn's disease at Groote Schuur Hospital during 1970–74. S. Afr. med. J. *49:* 693–697 (1975).

9   Hellers, G.: Crohn's disease in Stockholm County 1955–74. A study of epidemiology, results of surgical treatment and long-term prognosis. Acta chir. scand. *490:* suppl., pp. 1–83 (1979).

10 Brahme, F.; Lindstrom. C.; Wenckert, A.: Crohn's disease in a defined population. An epidemiological study of incidence, prevalence, mortality, and secular trends in the city of Malmö, Sweden, Gastroenterology *69:* 342–351 (1975).

11 Gilat, T.; Kuhn, R.; Gelman, E.; Mizrahy, O.: Lactase deficiency in Jewish communities in Israel. Am. J. dig. Dis. *15:* 895–904 (1970).

12 Tandon, R.; Mandell, H.; Spiro, H. M.; Thayer, W. R.; Jr.: Lactose intolerance in Jewish patients with ulcerative colitis. Am. J. dig. Dis. *16:* 845–848 (1971).

13 Leichter, J.: Lactose tolerance in a Jewish population. Am. J. dig. Dis. *16:* 1123–1126 (1971).

14 Rozen, P.; Zonis, J.; Yekutiel, P.; Gilat, T.: Crohn's disease in the Jewish population of Tel-Aviv Yafo. Epidemiological and clinical aspects. Gastroenterology *76:* 25–30 (1979).

15 Goodman, M. R.: Genetic disorders among Jewish people (Johns Hopkins University Press, Baltimore 1979).

16 Mourant A. E.; Kopec A. C.; Domaniewska-Sobezak, K.: Genetics of the Jews (Clarendon Press, Oxford 1978).

17 Gilat, T.: Lactase deficiency. The world pattern today. Israel J. med. Scis *15:* 369–373 (1979).

T. Gilat, MD, Department of Gastroenterology, Ichilov Hospital,
Tel-Aviv 64239 (Israel)

Front. gastrointest. Res., vol. 11, pp. 141–145 (Karger, Basel 1986)

Crohn's Disease in Specialised Groups

John Francis Mayberry

Queens Medical Centre, University Hospital of Nottingham, UK

Study of people with a significantly increased incidence of disease is of particular value in identifying possible aetiological factors. Inflammatory bowel disease is no exception and interest has recently focused on three groups – nurses and doctors, dietitians, and Mormons. Various aspects of their life-styles have encouraged studies of prevalence of inflammatory bowel disease. Medical personnel are exposed to many patients with these diseases and if they are transmissible then doctors and nurses are likely to have a higher prevalence than other people. Dietitians and Mormons have particular interests in diet and it has been suggested that diet and smoking habits may play a part in the development of inflammatory bowel disease.

Doctors and Nurses [1–3]

One of the earliest studies amongst doctors was conducted by *Goodman* et al. [1]. They reviewed 988 members of the American Gastroenterological Association and identified 8 cases of inflammatory bowel disease, giving a prevalence of $810/10^5$ population. This increased prevalence amongst doctors was attributed to an increased diagnostic awareness and it was also felt likely that a number of people with inflammatory bowel disease might be attracted to the profession. Two [1, 2] antibody studies have also failed to provide any support for an infective aetiology.

The possibility that Crohn's disease is infectious has often excited attention and although many attempts to transmit the disease to animals have been unsuccessful there have often been difficulties with the experimental laboratory animals used in these studies. It was against this background that we conducted a retrospective survey of nurses with inflammatory bowel disease [3] to see if those with Crohn's disease had had any greater exposure to diseased patients. Nurses are often in intimate contact with patients, their fomites and faeces and are at increased risk of certain diseases.

Nurses with inflammatory bowel disease were identified through the columns of the three major British nursing journals – Nursing Times, Nursing Mirror and Nursing Standard. One hundred and seven nurses with Crohn's disease and 70 with ulcerative colitis were asked to complete a detailed questionnaire about their nursing activities prior to the development of their illness. Of the 177 nurses with inflammatory bowel disease, 149 developed the condition after the start of training. A similar percentage of both groups of nurses had worked regularly with patients with inflammatory bowel disease prior to their own diagnosis (46% of those with Crohn's disease and 45% with ulcerative colitis). There is no support for the view that nurses can be infected with Crohn's disease by their patients.

There are about 300,000 qualified nurses in active employment in Britain. In our survey we identified 91 such nurses which gives a prevalence of about 29.3 cases/10^5. This figure is surprisingly similar to the prevalence reported from Nottingham and Aberdeen. Postal surveys may underestimate the prevalence of a disease and further studies of the frequency with which these diseases occur in nurses may be of value.

Dietitians [4]

In recent years interest has focused on the role of diet in the aetiology of Crohn's disease and there is considerable support for the observation that patients with Crohn's disease have an increased intake of sugar compared with controls. Differences in fibre consumption vary significantly from study to study and there is no clear indication as to its role. There have been several studies of dietary modification, but as yet little work has been done on the role of diet in preventing the appearance of inflammatory bowel disease. Are vegans at less risk of developing Crohn's disease or ulcerative colitis? Seventh Day Adventists avoid certain foods and have a low incidence of colonic cancer, but what about ulcerative colitis?

Table I. Frequency (%) of some gastrointestinal diseases amongst dietitians

Disease	Dietitians	General population
Appendicitis	12.3	12
Crohn's disease	0.1	0.06
Ulcerative colitis	0.3	0.08
Anorexia nervosa	1.7	0.1–0.5

With this in mind we undertook a survey of dietitians who were members of the British Dietetic Association. It seemed likely that a group with a professional interest in diet would follow a 'healthy' diet high in fibre and low in refined carbohydrates. Fifteen hundred questionnaires about gastrointestinal diseases including appendicitis, Crohn's disease and ulcerative colitis, peptic ulcer and anorexia nervosa were sent to members. Seven hundred and sixty replies were returned with a response rate of 51% (table I).

Only 3 dietitians had inflammatory bowel disease and these numbers are too small to allow adequate statistical analysis, but there is no indication that they are at less risk of developing inflammatory bowel disease.

Mormons [5, 6]

Members of the Church of Latter Day Saints or Mormons first appeared in the USA in the last century. They are of particular interest because of dietary prohibitions given in their 'Word of Wisdom'. Tobacco, alcohol, coffee, tea and addictive drugs are prohibited and a well-balanced diet including fresh food, vegetables and whole grain products is recommended. Although they have been present in Great Britain for many years their growth has become spectacular in recent decades and they are now said to have 100,000 members throughout the country.

The church is highly structured and church leaders were asked to identify who had Crohn's disease or ulcerative colitis and to record the active as well as the total membership of each church. The distinction between active and total membership is important as many members do not attend the church regularly and are also unlikely to follow dietary rules. Patients were subsequently sent a confidential questionnaire about date of diagnosis and its relationship to church membership.

Table II. Prevalence of inflammatory bowel disease in Mormons

Disease	Prevalence (cases/10^5 population)
Crohn's disease	79
Ulcerative colitis	389

Two hundred and thirty of the 342 branches in Britain reported details of membership and diseased members. The total membership was 56,650 but only 17,700 were active members who attended church regularly. Estimates of the prevalence of Crohn's disease and ulcerative colitis are based on the smaller figure, which more closely represents the population surveyed. There were 14 cases of Crohn's disease and 69 of ulcerative colitis reported (table II).

Six of the 14 patients with Crohn's disease completed a questionnaire; the average age at the time of diagnosis was 28 years and this was after a mean interval of 10 years of church membership. Twenty of the 69 patients with ulcerative colitis also completed a questionnaire. The mean age of the patients at the time of diagnosis was 33 years and 16 of the patients were diagnosed after a mean interval of 7 years as members of the church, suggesting that the high prevalence of the disease in Mormons is not due to ill people becoming converts.

The prevalence of Crohn's disease is similar to that reported in some other British studies, but ulcerative colitis was about 5 times more common than in Oxford and 3 times greater than in Copenhagen. Ulcerative colitis is twice as common as Crohn's disease, but in Mormons it is 5 times as common and Mormons seem to be at an increased risk of ulcerative colitis. Active Mormons are less likely to smoke than the rest of the population and those who do, smoke fewer cigarettes. It is of some interest that non-smokers appear to be at 3 times the risk of colitis and that ulcerative colitis is about 4 times more common in Mormons who largely abstain from smoking.

These preliminary results suggest that further studies should be conducted amongst Mormons and Adventists. Mornmons seem to be at an increased risk of developing ulcerative colitis, but none of the groups studied show a greater risk of developing Crohn's disease.

General Discussion

The incidence of Crohn's disease has increased since World War II. Initially, it was seen in North-Western Europe and North America. However, in recent years it has been seen with increasing frequency in Southern Europe, amongst immigrant groups and in developing countries. All of these features encourage us to look for specific aetiological factors. Laboratory research has covered the fields of infection and immunological abnormalities. Further clues may be obtained by epidemiological studies, and the consideration of social groups with distinct dietary or behavioural patterns may be of considerable value.

Japanese immigrants in the USA have not yet been the subject of research in this area. In Japan, Crohn's disease appears to be a very unusual condition, but nothing is known of its frequency in first and second generation Japanese Americans. Adventists have a particularly strict dietary code and there are sufficient of them in the USA to make epidemiological studies worthwhile. Occupational groups in the cigarette industry may provide insight into the role of tobacco in inflammatory bowel disease.

A number of studies have defined the incidence and prevalence of inflammatory bowel disease. Further studies need to consider groups with habits which may predispose them to ulcerative colitis or Crohn's disease.

References

1   Goodman, M. J.; Strickland, R. G.; Kirsner, J. B.: Inflammatory bowel disease and lymphocytotoxic antibody in members of the American Gastroenterological Association. Gastroenterology 76: 1140 (1979).
2   Mayberry, J. F.; Rhodes, J.; Matthews, N.; Wensinck, F.: Serum antibodies to anaerobic coccoid rods in patients with Crohn's disease or ulcerative colitis and in medical and nursing staff. Br. med. J. 282: 108 (1981).
3   Mayberry, J. F.; Newcombe, R. G.: Are nurses at an increased risk of developing inflammatory bowel disease? Digestion 22: 150–154 (1981).
4   Morgan, G. J.; Mayberry, J. F.: Common gastrointestinal diseases and anorexia nervosa in British dietitians. Publ. Hlth 97: 166–169 (1983).
5   Penny, W. J.; Penny, E.; Mayberry, J. F.; Rhodes, J.: Mormons, smoking and ulcerative colitis. Lancet ii: 1315 (1983).
6   Penny, W. J.; Penny, E.; Mayberry, J. F.; Rhodes, J.: Prevalence of inflammatory bowel disease among Mormons in Britain and Ireland. Soc. Sci. Med. 21: 287–290.

John Francis Mayberry, MD, MRCP, Queens Medical Centre, University Hospital of Nottingham, Nottingham NG7 2UH (UK)

Front. gastrointest. Res., vol. 11, pp. 146–154 (Karger, Basel 1986)

Smoking and Inflammatory Bowel Disease

Richard F. A. Logan, Kevin W. Somerville, Margaret Edmond,
Michael J. S. Langman

Departments of Community Health and Therapeutics, University of Nottingham,
Queen's Medical Centre, Nottingham, UK

Introduction

Non-smoking was first reported to be associated with ulcerative colitis (UC) by *Harries* et al. [1] in 1982 and the association has since been confirmed in several other studies [2–5]. However, as yet it has not been possible to determine whether this unexpected association precedes or follows the development of UC as it seems possible that non-smoking might be a consequence of developing any chronic disease. In contrast, smoking and Crohn's disease (CD) has been little studied. In Cardiff, CD patients were found to have similar smoking habits to those of a control group recruited from a fracture clinic but this finding has been difficult to interpret because of a poor response from the CD patients and the use of controls whose smoking habits are possibly unrepresentative of the general population. We have, therefore, carried out two case control studies enquiring about smoking habits in patients with UC and CD and compared them with community controls selected from the records of general practitioners (family doctors).

Patients and Methods

Both case series included all patients with UC and CD from a defined group of 52 general practices who were attending (77%) or had attended (23%) the City Hospital, Nottingham. The hospital case records of the 206 patients were reviewed to confirm a diagnosis of UC (124) or CD (82). Details of the patients are given in table I.

Table I. Case details

	Ulcerative colitis	Crohn's disease
Number of patients	124	82
Mean age (year) at diagnosis (range)	36 (12–75)	31 (10–73)
Current mean age	46	39
Male/female	58/66	29/53
Extent of disease		
Left colon	73	–
Total colon	47	–
Small bowel only	–	14
Large bowel only	–	25
Large and small bowel	–	43
Uncertain	4	–
Multiple attacks	114	71
Colectomy or bowel resection	23	45
Positive biopsy or histology report available[1]	114	56

[1] In some cases this information had been obtained at other hospitals before referral to the City Hospital

As part of the British National Health Service 98% of the population registers with a general practitioner (family doctor), which makes it possible to identify community controls from the records of general practitioners as follows. Each patient was matched with 2 controls, who were chosen by visiting the practitioner and using the practitioner's records or age and sex register to select the next 2 people alphabetically of the same sex and age within two years. Whenever possible, 2 reserve controls were taken in case selected controls had moved house or died but reserves were not otherwise used. Before we approached the controls the general practitioners were asked if there were medical or other reasons for not approaching them; the controls were not necessarily currently attending their doctor but were simply registered there.

Patients and controls were sent similar covering letters and a two-page questionnaire with general questions about family size, occupation, marital status and intake of tea, coffee and alcohol on the first page and enquiry that past and present smoking habits on the second page. If no reply was returned after 6–8 weeks, a second letter and questionnaire was posted and in the CD study a third reminder was posted after a further 8 weeks to any remaining non-responders.

Analysis. Smoking was arbitrarily defined as smoking more than 5 cigarettes, 3 cigars or 14 g (½ oz) of pipe tobacco weekly for at least 1 year. For patients, smoking habit at onset of disease was taken to be the habit reported 3 months before the onset of clinical disease; the smoking habit at the equivalent age was examined in the controls. To preserve the matched design of the study we used Miettinen's method for matched triplets, which permit analysis of complete and incomplete matched sets [6, 7]. For other analyses we used the chi-squared test with Yates correction and unpaired Student's t test.

Table II. Distributions of smoking habit

	% men		% women		Relative risk for smokers (M and F combined)	95% confidence limits	χ^2
	cases	controls	cases	controls			
Crohn's disease	(n=29)	(n=41)	(n=52)	(n=95)			
Ever smoked	75	65	72	38	4.0	1.9–8.1	14.2*
Current smokers	62	37	51	21	3.5	1.8–6.6	14.9*
Smoked at disease onset	65	45	63	24	4.8	2.4–9.7	21.0*
Ulcerative colitis	(n=56)	(n=88)	(n=64)	(n=113)			
Ever smoked	75	80	41	49	0.71	0.42–1.3	1.1
Current smokers	18	50	11	33	0.26	0.14–0.5	20.3*
Smoked at disease onset	20	64	17	37	0.16	0.08–0.33	32.8*

* $p < 0.001$.

Table III. Smoking at disease onset by social class

Social class	Cases			Controls		
	n	%	% smoking at onset	n	%	% smoking at onset
Crohn's disease						
I and II	19	22	74	29	21	24
III	47	58	62	73	54	37
IV and V	13	16	67	25	18	28
Not known	2	4		9	7	
Ulcerative colitis						
I and II	30	25	20	48	24	42
III	68	58	16	94	47	54
IV and V	17	14	18	43	21	56
Not known	3	3		16	8	

Results

Of the 206 patients approached, 3 were found to have left the area and 2 did not reply. Of the 412 controls approached, 337 (82%) replied. There were 138 complete case-control sets and in 55 sets the case and 1 control replied: these were used for the matched analysis.

The percentage distribution of smoking habits among patients and controls is shown in table II. The relative risks (RR) for a current smoker were 0.26 and 3.5 for UC and CD, respectively. Crohn's disease patients were less likely to be lifelong non-smokers than controls and although there was a tendency for the converse to occur in colitis, this was not significant. The pattern of UC patients being non-smokers and CD patients being smokers, was similar for men and women (for UC RR in smokers – men 0.25, women 0.27; for CD RR for smokers – men 3.0, women 3.9).

Smoking at Disease Onset

As a result of difficulty defining the clinical onset of CD in 3 patients it was not possible to determine the smoking pattern 3 months before onset and so they were excluded from the estimates of relative risk. CD patients were more likely to be smokers than control subjects at that corresponding age with a relative risk of 4.8: that for UC was 0.16.

Table IV. Relative risk of smoking at onset: disease distributions and histopathological findings

	Number of cases	Relative risk	95% confidence limits
Crohn's disease			
Small bowel only	14	3.5	0.8–14.6
Large bowel only	25	4.7	1.4–16.1
Large and small bowel	43	4.5	1.8–11.5
Granulomas	32	5.2	1.7–15.4
Transmural inflammation (no granulomas)	24	4.2	1.2–15.5
Ulcerative colitis			
Proctosigmoid	47	0.043	0.007–0.28
Disease to splenic flexure/transverse colon	26	0.11	0.014–0.83
Total colon affected	38	0.28	0.1–0.71

When smoking at disease onset only was considered, there were some differences in the pattern between men and women. In CD women were more likely to have been smokers before onset compared with controls than men compared with their controls, the relative risks being 8.2 for women compared to 2.7 for men but these differences were not statistically significant. In contrast the protection apparently afforded by smoking in UC was greater for men (RR = 0.08) than women (RR = 0.28) but this difference was also not significant.

Other Aspects of Smoking

Few patients or controls smoked cigars or a pipe and relative risk estimates for cigarette smoking alone were not significantly different whether cigar or pipe smokers were disregarded or included as non-smokers. Although the matching did not take social class into account the social class distributions, according to the Registrar General's classification, were similar (table III) and the excess or deficiency of smokers amongst the CD and UC patients, respectively, were seen across all social classes. None of the 62 ulcerative colitis patients who smoked or had smoked thought that smoking had a beneficial effect: the majority (56) thought that smoking had no effect and 6 gave no answer. Some other aspects of smoking and disease are given in tables IV and V. The trend for less extensive colitis to be associated with non-smoking was not significant (table IV). Crohn's patients on average stopped smoking later than their age and sex matched controls (table V).

Table V. Aspects of smoking in cases and controls

	Crohn's disease		Ulcerative colitis	
	Cases	Controls	Cases	Controls
Reported age of starting smoking, year				
Men	16.4	16.7	17.0	16.0
Women	17.7	18.2	17.9	18.4
Reported age of stopping smoking, year				
Men	45.0	25.5	36.1	42.2
Women	36.8	32.0	34.1	33.5
Reported maximum quantity of cigarettes smoked per day for a year				
Men	27	20	22	22
women	15	16	15	18
Reported quanitity of cigarettes currently smoked per day				
Men	18	13	15	18
women	12	13	9	16

Stopping Smoking in Relation to Disease Onset

Forty-two of the 55 ulcerative colitis subjects who stopped smoking had done so at least 3 months before the onset of symptoms. To assess the possibility that giving up smoking induces UC, table VI compares smokers and ex-smokers with never-smokers as the reference group. Protection from UC is still present amongst smokers but it does appear that ex-smokers may be at increased risk of developing UC.

In CD the number of ex-smokers at disease onset was small and although the RR suggests giving up smoking is associated with reduced risk of CD the 95% confidence limits are wide.

Discussion

We have found that patients with ulcerative colitis are less likely and those with Crohn's disease more likely to be smokers than age and sex matched controls drawn from the community [8, 9]. These differences antedated the onset of both diseases and were independent of social class. As the association of ulcerative colitis with non-smoking has now been

Table VI. Relative risk[1] at disease onset for current smokers and ex-smokers

	Cases	Controls	Relative risk	95% confidence limits
Crohn's disease				
Never smoked	24	78	1.0	
Ex-smokers	5	14	1.2	0.38–3.6
Current smokers	52	41	4.2	2.3–7.7
Total	81	133[2]		
Ulcerative colitis				
Never smoked	52	76	1.0	
Ex-smokers	46	24	2.8	1.54–5.1
Current smokers	22	99	0.32	0.18–0.57
Total	120	199[2]		

[1] Estimates based on unmatched analysis.
[2] In some controls smoking state at onset was uncertain.

shown in at least five different studies, the possibility of a chance association can be dismissed [1–5]. A deficit of lung cancer and deaths from cardiovascular disease amongst colitics is also consistent with a real association [10]. In contrast, the findings for patients with Crohn's disease have not been previously reported. While no single study can exclude the possibility of a chance association the estimated relative risks are large, with accordingly small p values. It also seems unlikely that the findings could be explained by some unidentified systematic bias in our method of enquiry. Both groups of patients were approached in the same way, with identical questionnaires, so that any tendency to under or over estimate smoking habits would be the same for both groups and would not reduce the associations demonstrated.

Harries et al. [1] in Cardiff found that the proportion of smokers amongst their Crohn's patients was similar to that amongst their control subjects. It seems possible that their study failed to detect a difference between Crohn's patients and controls because they used patients attending fracture clinics as controls, of whom 44% were smokers. Furthermore, the response rate from the Crohn's patients was low and it may be that non-responders are more likely to be smokers. The reported smoking habits of our controls were similar to those found in recent national data where 38% of men and 32% of women reported themselves as smokers [11]!

The finding in our study that stopping smoking was associated with an increased risk of UC was unexpected and difficult to explain. Previous studies were unable to assess smoking at disease onset and the small increase in risk for ex-smokers [1, 2] that they demonstrated, could be explained by patients stopping smoking after the onset of UC. Clearly, the association with ex-smoking needs confirmation and until this is obtained we are inclined to treat it as only a chance finding [12].

Possible explanations for the differences in smoking habit between the two types of inflammatory bowel disease are still highly speculative. Those who favour psychosomatic factors in the aetiology of ulcerative colitis, might suggest that smoking behaviour is evidence of a predisposed personality type. While there is some evidence that psychosomatic factors may play a part in ulcerative colitis, the evidence is contradictory and psychosomatic factors have not been considered to have a role in Crohn's disease [13]. So little is known of the effect of smoking on colonic function or other aspects of gastrointestinal function, that it is difficult to suggest a direct mechanism. Possibilities include changes in bowel motility or in susceptibility to various pathogens. Smoking is known to produce complex changes in immune function [14, 15].

As cigarette smoking is associated with an increased consumption of refined sugar [16, 17], smoking may explain the association of refined sugar consumption and Crohn's disease which has been previously reported [18, 22]. As no association has been found between sugar consumption and ulcerative colitis it is likely that the associations with smoking habits are the primary relationships.

In conclusion, there is no explanation why Crohn's disease tends to occur more commonly in smokers and ulcerative colitis more commonly in non-smokers. These two associations are, however, consistent with the hypothesis of a genetic predisposition to inflammatory bowel disease with smoking habit determining which of the two diseases develops. Other factors besides smoking must play a role in the development of Crohn's disease; smoking cannot account for the occurrence of the disease in children. Nevertheless, an association of Crohn's disease with smoking might partly account for the emergence of this disease during the 20th century.

References

1   Harries, A. D.; Baird, A.; Rhodes, J.: Non-smoking. A feature of ulcerative colitis. Br. med. J. *284:* 706 (1982).
2   Jick, H.; Walker, A. M.: Cigarette smoking and ulcerative colitis. New Engl. J. Med. *308:* 261–263 (1983).

3 Bures, J.; Fixa, B.; Komarkova, O.; Fingerland, A.: Non-smoking. A feature of ulcerative colitis. Br. med. J. *285:* 440 (1982).

4 Gyde, S. N.; Prior, P.; Taylor, K.; Allan, R. N.: Cigarette smoking, blood pressure and ulcerative colitis. Gut *24:* A998 (1983).

5 Holdstock, G.; Savage, D.; Harman, M.; Wright, R.: Should patients with inflammatory bowel disease smoke? Br. med. J. *288:* 362 (1984).

6 Miettinen, O. S.: Estimation of relative risk from individually matched series. Biometrics *26:* 75–86 (1970).

7 Breslow, N. E.; Day, N. E.: Statistical methods in cancer research. Vol. I. The analysis of case-control studies (International Agency for Research on Cancer, Lyons 1980).

8 Logan, R. F. A.; Edmond, M.; Somerville, K. W.; Langman, M. J. S.: Smoking and ulcerative colitis. Br. med. J. *288:* 751–753 (1984).

9 Somerville, K. W.; Logan, R. F. A.; Edmond, M.; Langman, M. J. S.: Smoking and Crohn's disease. Br. med. J. *289:* 954–956 (1984).

10 Gyde, S. N.; Prior, P.; Dew, M. J.; Saunders, V.; Waterhouse, J. A. H.; Allan, R. N.: Mortality in ulcerative colitis. Gastroenterology *83:* 36–43 (1982).

11 Office of Population Censuses and Surveys: Cigarette smoking: 1972 to 1982 (HMSO, London 1983).

12 Logan, R. F. A.; Langman, M. J. S.: Smoking and ulcerative colitis (Letter). Br. med. J. *288:* 1307 (1984).

13 Helzer, J. E.; Stillings, W. A.; Chammas, S.; Norland, C. C.; Alpers, D. H.: A controlled study of the association between ulcerative colitis and psychiatric diagnoses. Dig. Dis. Sci. *27:* 513–518 (1982).

14 Ferson, M.; Edwards, A.; Lind, A.; Milton, G. N.; Hersey, P.: Lower natural killer cell activity and immunoglobulin levels associated with smoking in human subjects. Int. J. Cancer *23:* 603–609 (1979).

15 Hersey, P.; Prendergast, D; Edwards, A.: Effects of smoking on the immune system: follow-up studies in normal subjects after cessation of smoking. Med. J. Aust. *ii:* 425–429 (1983).

16 Bennett, A. E.; Doll, R.; Howell, R. W.: Sugar consumption and cigarette smoking. Lancet *i:* 1011–1014 (1970).

17 Elwood, P. C.; Waters, W. E.; Moore, S.; Sweetnam, P.: Sucrose consumption and ischaemic heart disease in the community. Lancet *i:* 1014–1016 (1970).

18 Martini, G. A.; Brandes, J. N.: Increased consumption of refined carbohydrate in patients with Crohn's disease. Klin. Wschr. *54:* 367–371 (1976).

19 Thornton, J. R.; Emmett, P. M.; Heaton, K. W.: Diet and Crohn's disease. Characteristics of the pre-illness diet. Br. med. J. *ii:* 762–764 (1979).

20 Kasper, H.; Sommer, H.: Dietary fibre and nutrient intake in Crohn's disease. Am. J. clin. Nutr. *32:* 1898–1901 (1979).

21 Mayberry, J. F.; Rhodes, J.; Newcombe, R. G.: Increased sugar consumption in Crohn's disease. Digestion *20:* 323–326 (1980).

22 Janerot, G.; Jarnmark, I.; Nilsson, K.: Consumption of refined sugar by patients with Crohn's disease, ulcerative colitis or irritable bowel syndrome. Scand. J. Gastroent. *18:* 999–1002 (1983).

Richard F. A. Logan, MD, Department of Community Health, The University of Nottingham, Queen's Medical Centre, Clifton Boulevard, Nottingham, NG7 2UH (UK)

Front. gastrointest. Res., vol. 11, pp. 155–157 (Karger, Basel 1986)

Smoking and Colitis

John Rhodes

Department of Gastroenterology, University Hospital of Wales, Health Park, Cardiff, UK

Introduction

Our initial observation that there appeared to be an association between ulcerative colitis and non-smoking was almost made by chance. Dr. *Harries* was investigating the nutritional status of patients with Crohn's disease and examining various anthropometric measurements which may help to identify those who were undernourished. The mid-arm circumference was one such measurement which was made on patients with Crohn's disease and control patients with ulcerative colitis as well as matched healthy subjects from the general population [1]. Since smoking affects weight, it was important to take into consideration the smoking habits of the patient groups and healthy controls. To our surprise, and annoyance, we were only able to identify 7 out of 106 patients with ulcerative colitis who were cigarette smokers. This made it difficult to compare the groups because of the disproportionately small number of smokers. We then realised that another way of looking at the data was to question whether the majority of patients with ulcerative colitis were non-smokers.

The Study

To examine this finding the study was extended using a postal questionnaire to ask 230 patients with ulcerative colitis and 192 patients with Crohn's disease about their smoking habits. The patients with ulcerative colitis were matched with 230 control subjects who were attending a Fracture Clinic [2].

Table I. Details of results from a postal questionnaire in patients with ulcerative colitis, matched healthy controls and patients with Crohn's disease

	Number of subjects	Current cigarette smokers, %	Subjects who have never smoked, %	Ex-smokers, %	Subjects from non-smoking households, %
Ulcerative colitis	230	8[1]	48[1]	40[1]	76[1]
Healthy controls	230	44	36	20	51
Crohn's disease	192	42	30	27	60

[1] These figures in patients with ulcerative colitis differ significantly from healthy controls.

Results

The current smoking habits for the three groups are given in table I and show that only 8 per cent with ulcerative colitis were current cigarette smokers; this confirmed our initial finding and was consistent for all age groups. This figure of 8% compared with 44% in our healthy controls and 42% in the patient group with Crohn's disease. These figures from the healthy controls were very similar to National figures from the United Kingdom obtained in a general household survey [3].

The non-smokers with ulcerative colitis were made up of significantly greater numbers who had either never smoked or were ex-smokers, compared with the other groups. Furthermore, a significant excess of patients also came from non-smoking households.

Discussion

We concluded in this initial study that a highly significant number of patients with ulcerative colitis are non-smokers and made up of those who have never smoked as well as ex-smokers. We were unable to identify any difference between the patients with Crohn's disease and our control group.

Since that time the finding has been confirmed in Czechoslavakia [4], the USA [5] and Nottingham [6]. The association of ulcerative colitis and non-smoking raises the possibility that smoking may exert a protective action against ulcerative colitis. There is, however, no direct evidence to support this. A few anecdotal reports have appeared in the literature recording the clinical history of patients who smoked and experienced a relapse of their colitis when they attempted to discontinue smoking and in one report Nicorette chewing gum was claimed to have a beneficial effect in maintaining remission [7, 8]. A more formal approach to identify patients with colitis who are smokers or have previously been smokers may be of value, for most smokers have attempted to discontinue the habit at some time and would, no doubt, have noticed a deterioration in their bowel symptoms during such stressful periods. Any protective effect of smoking or nicotine is potentially of great interest because of the possible new therapeutic approaches which could develop from further investigation.

References

1   Harries, A. D.; Baird, A.; Rhodes, J.: Non-smoking: a feature of ulcerative colitis. Br. med. J. *284:* 706 (1982).
2   Harries, A. D.; Jones, L.; Heatley, R. V.; Rhodes, J.: Smoking habits and inflammatory bowel disease: effect on nutrition. Br. med. J. *284:* 1161 (1982).
3   Capell, P. J.: Trends in cigarette smoking in the United Kingdom. Health Trends *10:* 49–54 (1978).
4   Bures, J.; Fixa, B.; Komarkova, O.; Fingerland, A.: Non-smoking. A feature of ulcerative colitis. Br. med. J. *285:* 440 (1982).
5   Jick, H.; Walker, A. M.; Cigarette smoking and ulcerative colitis. New Engl. J. Med. *308:* 261–263 (1983).
6   Logan, R.; Edmund, M.; Langman, M. J. S.: Is non-smoking associated with ulcerative colitis (Abstract) Gut *24:* A499 (1983).
7   De Castella, H.: Non-smoking. A feature of ulcerative colitis. Br. med. J. *284:* 1706 (1982).
8   Roberts, C. J.; Diggle, R.: Non-smoking: a feature of ulcerative colitis. Br. med. J. *285:* 440 (1982).

John Rhodes, MD, FRCP, Department of Gastroenterology, University Hospital of Wales, Heath Park, Cardiff CF4 4XW (UK)

Front. gastrointest. Res., vol. 11, pp. 158–176 (Karger, Basel 1986)

Environmental Factors in Inflammatory Bowel Disease[1]

T. Gilat[a], *M. J. S. Langman*[b], *P. Rozen*[a]

[a] Department of Gastroenterology, Ichilov Hospital and Tel Aviv University Sackler Faculty of Medicine, Tel Aviv, Israel; [b] Department of Therapeutics, University Hospital, Nottingham, UK

The etiology of ulcerative colitis (UC) and Crohn's disease (CD) is unknown. We are not even certain whether their grouping under the heading of inflammatory bowel disease (IBD) is pathogenetically justified and it is just as possible that we are dealing with more than two diseases. In this situation it is worthwhile to examine the evidence accumulated from epidemiologic studies and observations relevant to etiology. A prime question to be considered is whether this evidence points to the predominance of environmental-exogenous factors or genetic-endogenous factors in the causation of the disease(s). We will review and summarize the data which, in our opinion, point to the major role played by environmental factors in the causation of the disease(s).

The Evidence for the Effect of Environmental Factors in IBD

Changing Incidence

Figure 1 shows the incidence of CD in the recent decades in Aberdeen [1], Baltimore [2], Basle [3], Cardiff [4], Copenhagen [5], Glasgow [6], Gothenburg [7], Malmo [8], Marburg [9], Minnesota [10], Nottingham [11], Stockholm [12], Uppsala [13], and Tel Aviv [14].

All the above were population studies including all, or almost all, the patients with CD in a defined geographical area. Only the study from Baltimore was based on hospitalized cases [2]. Only the initial and last incidence in each study area are shown in figure 1. It is readily apparent that the incidence of CD rose very sharply (by several hundred percent) in all these areas in recent decades.

[1] The International Cooperative Study of 'Childhood Factors in IBD' was supported in part by a grant from the National Foundation for Ileitis and Colitis (USA).

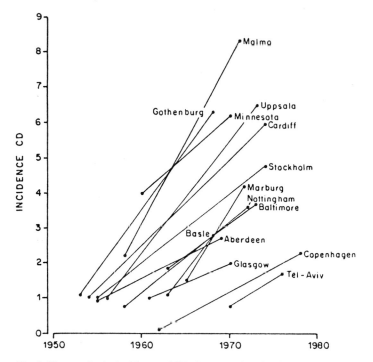

Fig. 1. Changes in the incidence of CD, in recent decades, in various geographical areas. Initial and last incidence are given for each study.

Interpretation of the time-trend curves is impeded by two important factors. Firstly, growing diagnostic awareness could contribute, at least in part, to the apparent increase in frequency of CD, and secondly with growing awareness there has been a tendency towards shortening of the interval between symptom onset and disease diagnosis. Figure 2 shows that the increase in recorded frequency of CD in Stockholm county is approximately 9% compound per annum [12]. The compound nature of the growth inevitably implies that after 10–20 years the absolute numbers of cases recorded each year have risen greatly.

Figure 3 shows the effects upon plotted chronological incidence data if true growth in incidence continues or stops and if shortening of the diagnostic interval continues or stops. Though the shape of the curve could be altered by the cessation of diagnostic shortening, such an effect would not persist and therefore could not account for a plateau in the growth curve which was maintained, although it would cause a temporary interruption.

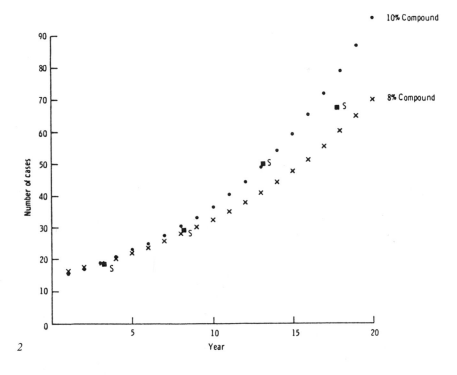

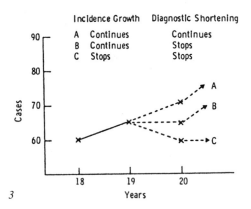

Fig. 2. Increasing frequency of CD in Stockholm County(S), compared with mathematical compound growth curves.

Fig. 3. Theoretical effects of changes in growth rates and in interval between onset and diagnosis of CD.

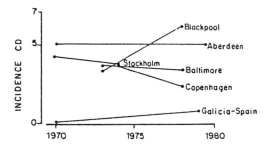

Fig. 4. Incidence of CD in recent years in several locations.

Deciding the precise contribution of increased diagnostic awareness is difficult. In recent years disease of the large bowel which was, for instance, segmental in nature has been likely to be described as Crohn's disease, whereas in the past it would probably have been categorized as ulcerative colitis. Generally, frequency rates of UC and CD differ somewhat, but not greatly. Therefore, if large numbers of patients were now being described as having CD where in the past they would have been called cases of UC, one would have expected a commensurate decrease in its frequency to match any rising frequency of CD. This does not seem to have occurred. Furthermore, the increased frequency of CD has been observed to include both small and large bowel disease.

Bias, due to freer access to medical facilities, was probably excluded in the UK and Scandinavian studies, where socialized medicine was available throughout that time. The rising incidence found in population studies is supported by rising mortality rates, despite improved medical management, and by higher rates for first hospital admissions [15]. All these data firmly support the contention that there has been a true and marked rise in the incidence of *CD*, in recent decades, in most industrialized countries. This trend may be changing. Figure 4 shows the incidence of CD in recent years in Aberdeen [16], Baltimore [2], Blackpool [17], Copenhagen [5], Galicia (Spain) [18], and Stockholm [12]. In most of these areas the incidence of CD seems to have reached a plateau and to have stopped rising. The data from Galicia may represent the rising incidence that is still occurring in areas where the process of industralization and urbanization is continuing.

The incidence of *UC* seems to have reached a plateau at an earlier period and has been stable, in recent decades, in most population studies. The data for Aberdeen [19], Baltimore [2], Cape Town [20], Copenhagen [5], Malmo [8], Marburg (FRG) [9], New Zealand [21], North Tees (UK) [22], Stockholm [23], Tel Aviv [24] and Hong Kong [27] are shown in figure 5. In Stockholm the incidence had been rising but has now reached

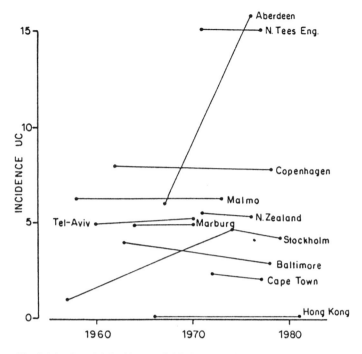

Fig. 5. Mostly stable incidence of UC, in recent decades, in several geographic areas.

a plateau. The only exception to this trend was a study from North-Eastern Scotland where the rise in incidence seems to have coincided with the establishment of a GI unit in that area [19]. It is noteworthy (fig. 4) that the highest incidence figures were reported from the UK and the lowest from Hong Kong which reflects the low incidence of IBD in developing populations.

Incidence in Developing Populations

While the incidence of UC and probably CD may have reached a plateau in industralized countries, with western cultural patterns of life, at least as judged by data from Western Europe and, perhaps, the USA, the incidence of both diseases seems to be rising sharply in some other populations. Judging correctly whether such changes are occurring is difficult for the following reasons. Many of the geographic areas where IBD was previously detected infrequently have been characterized by having high frequencies of infective dysenteric illnesses and by poorly developed

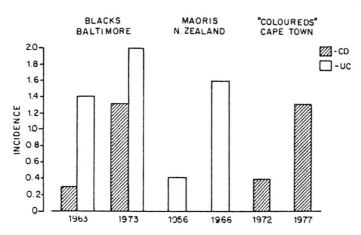

Fig. 6. Rising incidence of both UC and CD in developing populations of different geographic areas, in recent decades.

health care services. Therefore, we cannot be sure whether the IBD, which is now being recognized, was previously present but unidentified.

These reservations cannot account for the low frequencies of IBD recorded in native-born Israelis, in Israelis of non-European origin [14], in white South Africans [20, 25] and in the Japanese [26]. Furthermore, the very sparse reports of IBD in, for instance, colored South Africans [20, 25], Hong Kong Chinese [27] and New Zealand Maoris [21, 28] seem very unlikely to be accounted for by the consistent misdiagnosis of chronic infective conditions such as tuberculosis and amoebiasis. The tendency for IBD to spare countries with a tropical or relatively warm climate, and in which coincidentally the process of industralization is still ongoing, is emphasized by low recorded frequencies of CD, a half or less of those in the United Kingdom, in Spain [18] and Italy [20].

The tendency for the IBD frequency distribution to be inversely related to that of acute infective dysenteries is unexplained. A protective effect through early contact with gut infection, seems possible. The rising incidence of both diseases in developing populations in Baltimore [2], Cape Town [20, 25] and New Zealand [28] is shown in figure 6.

Studies in Migrants

A classical epidemiologic method to demonstrate the causative effect of environmental factors in a disease process has been the study of migrants from low- to high-incidence areas. There have been recent reports of IBD occurring in migrants to the UK, from various developing areas [30, 31]. These studies lack quantitative data on the incidence of

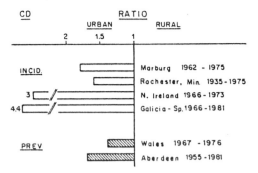

Fig. 7. A higher incidence and prevalence of CD in urban as compared to rural residents.

IBD both in the migrants to the UK as well as in their countries of origin. There are, however, solid quantitative epidemiologic data for one group of migrants in various parts of the world, namely Ashkenazi Jews. These are detailed in another chapter [32]. The data show a very marked variation in the incidence of both CD and UC in Jews, in various parts of the world, paralleling the incidence of these diseases in the general population of the study areas. However, the incidence in the Jewish population, in each area, was greater than that in the non-Jews living in the same areas [32].

Studies of changes in disease frequency in migrant populations are of value, not only because they help to distinguish between genetic and environmental contributions to disease frequency, but also because they can provide clues to the critical time periods which influence disease occurrence. Thus, migrant studies in IBD could be used to determine whether the timing of the move, in infancy, childhood or adult life, affected the development of IBD and whether a particular duration of stay in the adopted country was necessary. Based on such information it might be possible to concentrate epidemiological searches in a more relevant manner.

Urban-Rural Differences
The incidence and prevalence of CD were determined in several population studies in urban and rural residents, of the same population, in the same time period. The data from Aberdeen [16], Galicia (Spain) [18], Marburg [9], North Ireland [33], Rochester, Minn. [10], and Wales [34], are shown in figure 7. It can be seen that the frequency of both diseases is higher in urban than in rural residents of the same population. The same trend was found whether measured in terms of prevalence or

incidence. The figure shows representative data from major, recent studies. With a few exceptions, similar results were found for UC and CD in some previous studies [12].

The lower disease frequency, in rural populations, could reflect poorer medical services or the reluctance of country dwellers to seek medical advice. The consistency of the trend towards raised urban: rural ratios does not, of itself, help in determining if urban populations are particularly exposed to factors causing IBD. In most areas differences are fairly small, with ratios of less than 2:1 when measured as incidence or prevalence. But the fact that the differences are detectable in areas with free health care gives some support to the belief that etiological factors are more prevalent in towns.

General Conclusions

Taken overall, the incidence patterns of IBD indicate that environmental influences prevalent in industrialized countries with western cultural patterns of life, have marked effects upon the liability to have IBD, whether CD or UC. The similarity of incidence and prevalence data in North Western Europe suggest that whatever factor or factors operate, they are equally and uniformly distributed. Whilst the limited information available from migrant studies indicates that these factors may still exert their effect in adult life.

Putative Pathogenic Factors in IBD

It is much easier to demonstrate that environmental factors are important in IBD than to identify these factors. Table I lists some suggested factors.

Dietary Factors

Since the intestinal wall forms a barrier between the milieu interieu and the exterior of the body, as expressed within the lumen of the gut, and inflammatory bowel disease has its main impact at the mucosal interface, it is natural to seek dietary factors which might influence the liability to have IBD.

Prospective studies of populations with known habits are impractical because IBD disease incidence rates are so low. It would require the identification of the dietary habits of enormous groups of people for enough cases of IBD to be identified to allow reliable comparative studies. Broad geographical comparisons are also impractical, because in general terms the frequency of IBD either varies very little, for instance between differ-

Table I. Suggested pathogenetic factors in IBD

Dietary
  Bottle-feeding, sugar and cereal consumption,
  dietary fiber, chemically modified fats

Infectious
  Transmissible agents, infantile gastroenteritis,
  delayed exposure (sheltered child)

Chemical
  Contraceptives, smoking

Psychosomatic

---

ent parts of Western Europe, or is largely unmeasured, though probably rare, for instance, in tropical Africa. Even if comparisons were to be attempted between areas of high frequency (Scandinavia and the United Kingdom) and areas of lower frequency (such as India or Africa), the dietary habits and general customs of the population groups would be so different in so many respects that no useful information would be likely to be generated.

Retrospective case control studies would therefore seem to be the only possible methods, but there are considerable and perhaps insurmountable difficulties which hinder them. Firstly, the incubation period of IBD is unknown and therefore if questions are to be asked we do not know whether they should be directed at periods 1, 2, 5 or 10 years (or even earlier) prior to symptom onset. Nor do we know if that period is fixed or varies from one person to another. Secondly, we cannot be sure that the development of the disease will not alter patients' perception of antecedent habits or tastes. Thus, if, for instance, diseased patients with a raised caloric requirement developed a tendency to eat more of all or particular nutrients, then it is conceivable, and even likely, that they would believe that their habits had never been otherwise. Thirdly, individual recall of previous diet is inevitably limited, and becomes more limited as time elapses after the period in which it is proposed to take an interest. Patients may also have unquantifiable tendencies to suggest that their pre-morbid habits were particularly healthy (or unhealthy). Thus, patients aware, as most must be in Western countries, of the current belief in the virtues of high fibre and low sugar diets, may give answers consonant with or in contradiction to these diets. A fourth difficulty arises in choosing controls, as in classical epidemiological work we seek to choose control individuals who are as similar as possible to the test group, but lack the specific disease in question. Such an equivalent disease group to IBD does not exist.

Despite these difficulties, investigators have carried out a large number of case-control studies in which infant and other feeding habits have been examined.

Lack of Breast-Feeding. The occurrence of IBD in Western populations has inevitably been associated with the tendency to bottle-feed rather than breast-feed. Over 20 years ago *Acheson and Truelove* [35] suggested that early weaning was associated with increased liability to have UC, and lately *Bergstrand and Hellers* [36] have brought forward evidence to suggest that CD is associated with a reduced duration of breast-feeding. However, a similar but less-detailed investigation by *Whorwell* et al. [37] failed to detect any suggestive trends for CD, although suggesting that a history of never having been breast-fed was associated with later liability to UC.

Deciding which, if any, of these sets of data have meaning is difficult. Thus, *Whorwell* et al. [37] questioned only the patients or controls, and not the parents, and the mean age of those questioned (37 years) was relatively high when one considers that if a history of deficient breast-feeding was significant, then the maximum impact might be expected to be in the occurrence of the disease in childhood. Furthermore, the numbers of patients questioned, 51 with UC and 57 with CD, were relatively small, reducing confidence in the meaning of differences, even if responses to questions were true measures of feeding habits nearly 40 years earlier. In contrast, 308 patients were questioned in Stockholm [36] and their habits were compared with those of controls matched for the same day of birth and district of Sweden. In addition, the information given was checked with that provided by parents or some other reliable source. In a recently conducted International Study (see below) the frequency of breast-feeding and its duration was not different in patients with IBD and controls.

Sugar Consumption. Patients with CD have consistently been found to give histories of greater average daily sugar consumption in the past than controls [38–43]. Judging the significance of this trend is difficult. Attempts were generally made to establish what the pre-morbid habits of the patients might have been, but the duration of disease in the patient groups studied was very variable, with a mean of 10 years symptoms in one set [40] and a range of 1–9 months (median 5 months) in another [41]. There must therefore be considerable doubt as to whether the histories elicited from patients, with disease of long standing, actually represented pre-morbid habits. Where duration of history was taken into account, *Thornton* et al. [41] found no difference in the average (high) sugar consumption in their patients when utilizing a division between symptom onset, more or less than 12 months earlier, in newly diagnosed cases. The reliability of data obtained following this subdivision may be fairly low given that an initial group of 30 patients were being divided into two subgroups. *Jarnerot* et al. [43] again found that sugar consumption was greater in CD patients than in controls, but noted that sugar consumption was not increased in the subgroup where diagnoses had been made less than 6 months before, suggesting that illness modified responses to questions.

Deciding whether any trend towards increased sugar consumption in Crohn's disease does indeed provide an etiological clue is difficult. In favor of the association are the consistency with which it has been detected, a failure to find a similar trend in patients with ulcerative colitis, and a failure to establish that CD patients have altered taste perception for sugar [44–46]. Against this association is the suggestion that the presence of disease did alter responses to questions, the difficulty of placing weight upon data collected about habits long in the past, often without any apparent attempt to question controls for matching periods. Even if an association is established it is not necessarily primary and causal. Thus, we already have evidence that CD patients are particularly likely to be smokers. Previous epidemiological studies of cardiovascular disease have shown that smoking and sugar consumption tend to be correlated, and it is therefore possible that any association between sugar intake and Crohn's disease is more directly related to smoking habits.

Dietary Fiber. It has also been suggested that dietary fibre deficiency predisposes to CD, but the data examining this possibility show no consistent trends [41, 42]. The general difficulties of deciding whether retrospective dietary analyses give true pictures of past habits, and the possibility that patients may have reduced fibre intake deliberately because of symptoms associated with bolus impaction in segments of diseased bowel, greatly impedes assessment.

Cereal Consumption. An increased cereal consumption in childhood was found in patients with IBD by some authors [47], but not by others [48, 49]. In a Multicenter International Study described later, no differences were found between patients and controls in relation to cereal consumption. Fruit and vegetable consumption was lower in patients than controls, but it could not be determined whether it followed or antedated the disease.

Modified Fats. It was recently suggested that chemically modified 'hardened' fats such as margarine are more often consumed by IBD patients [50]. The data are based mainly on estimated margarine/butter consumption ratios in various countries in relation to the incidence of IBD in the same countries. More precise and better controlled studies are needed to substantiate or refute this hypothesis.

Infectious Factors

Transmissible Agents. The search for infectious agents in CD and UC is almost as old as the history of these diseases. Bacteria, viruses, chlamydia, L forms, etc. have all been suspected and intensively investigated. Various animal transmission studies have been performed and cytopathic effects or the induction of lymphoma in experimental animal systems have been claimed. The data have recently been reviewed [51, 52] and a detailed description is beyond the scope of this article. Suffice it to say that intensive search has not so far yielded conclusive results.

Theoretically, there are several possibilities. Firstly, contagion with a pathogen which is slow to grow would account for the indolent nature of most IBD and for difficulties of its culture. Secondly, exposure to a pathogen which results in permanently altered tissue responsiveness to what in other healthy individuals would be insignificant stresses, could explain the many immunological manifestations in IBD. Thirdly, exposure to a pathogenic stress which is ordinarily overcome quickly and with ease might in specific circumstances lead to long continued disease, perhaps with a considerable latent interval.

Sheltered Child. This hypothesis is in some ways the opposite of the infectious hypothesis. Instead of being exposed to a rare infectious agent invading the diseased bowel and causing disease, the child with IBD is assumed to be over-sheltered and to be exposed to a common infectious agent later in life than other children. This delayed exposure may trigger a different and inappropriate immunologic response, causing IBD. This is similar to paralytic polio affecting more frequently sheltered, well-to-do children, while children of lower socioeconomic classes come in contact with the virus at an earlier age and develop immunity. It is also similar to the hypothesis that Hodgkin's disease is caused by a delayed exposure to the EB virus [53]. There are, at present, no firm data to prove or refute the sheltered child hypothesis.

Epidemiological methods are difficult to apply. Conventional, though complicated, mathematical clustering techniques can be used to determine if patients are in the right place at the right time to become infected and to infect each other [54]. Difficulties arise in several ways; firstly, we have no means of judging what duration or form of contact would be necessary. The general lack of husband and wife pairs with disease and the absence of IBD developing in doctors and nurses treating these patients, argues against significant infectivity once disease is expressed. Secondly, clustering analyses have in fact shown no evidence of case aggregation as judged within space by domicile or place of work, or within time. However, whether the forms of contact examined were indeed relevant is impossible to determine, thus contact through the use of common sports facilities might be more important than living in the same street or working in the same factory.

Other approaches to be considered include analyses of the types of 'trivial' infective illness suffered in the past by patients, and considering the general patterns of diseases within patients' families, and of general illness suffered by patients themselves.

Infective Gastroenteritis. Whorwell et al. [37] suggested that a history of infantile gastroenteritis was significantly more common in patients with IBD than in controls, and postulated that this early insult predisposed the bowel to subsequent disease. Whether recall of previous histories by patients (and controls) unchecked by reference to parents, and covering time periods several decades before would be likely to be accurate, must be doubted. Furthermore, the case series were rather small. If gastroenteritis were more common in infancy it could be a secondary phenomenon, for instance associated with bottle-feeding rather than breast-feeding.

Chemical Factors

Contraceptives. Isolated case reports suggested that women who used oral contraceptives might be prone to develop colonic Crohn's disease. Rhodes et al. [55] found that 10 out of 16 women with CD, confined to the colon, had taken oral contraceptives, compared with 12 of 49 with small intestinal disease and 3 out of 35 with ulcerative colitis. They also suggested that nongranulomatous disease of the colon, in particular, might remit for prolonged periods when oral contraceptive treatment ceased. The authors correlated their findings with a possible tendency for colonic CD to be particularly common in women. Confirmatory data, or otherwise, should be reasonably easy to obtain by reference to the comprehensive records maintained about the health of many thousands of women practicing different methods of contraception. They, in effect, supply a cohort which can be prospectively studied from the date of entry to their contraception surveillance studies.

Table II. Childhood factors in IBD—International Cooperative Study

Participating centers
Chicago (USA), University of Chicago School of Medicine
Cleveland (USA), Cleveland Clinic
Copenhagen (Denmark), Herlev Hospital
Genova (Italy), National Institute for Research of Cancer
Leiden (The Netherlands), University Hospital
Liverpool (UK), Broadgreen Hospital
Lyon (France), Lyon Medical Center
New Haven (USA), Yale University School of Medicine
New York (USA), Lenox Hill Hospital
Nice (France), Hôpital de Cimiez
Nottingham (UK), University Hospital
Orebro (Sweden), Central County Hospital
Tel Aviv (Israel), Tel Aviv University, Ichilov Hospital
Toronto (Canada), Toronto General Hospital

Smoking. Several recent studies have reported that nonsmokers were significantly more frequent among patients with UC than among matched controls [56–58]. This was even more marked at onset of UC and was accounted for mainly by patients who had stopped smoking [58]. It was even suggested that smoking or nicotine might be therapeutically effective in UC. Interestingly, smokers were more frequent among patients with CD than UC [56, 59] or controls [59]. It was suggested that among subjects predisposed to IBD, smokers might preferentially develop CD while nonsmokers might develop UC [59]. The subject is intriguing and more direct studies of this unusual association are awaited.

Psychosomatic Factors

These were in vogue a few decades ago. Specific personality traits could not be demonstrated in patients with UC or CD. Present-day medical opinion holds that psychological attitudes and disturbances, occasionally found in these patients, are the result and not the cause of the disease [60].

Current Research

In view of the evidence that environmental factors are important in IBD and the difficulty in identifying them in small-scale studies, a large-scale International Cooperative Study was recently performed. Since IBD most frequently starts in the 2nd and 3rd decades, the study included only patients whose disease began before age 20. To obtain reliable information, only patients whose present age was below 25 and whose mother was alive were included. Since large numbers of suitable patients and controls were required and geographic-environmental variability was considered an asset, the study was carried out in 14 centers (table II) in 9 countries, using uniform questionnaires. Two age- and sex-matched controls were studied for each patient having either UC or CD. One control was a patient with minor gastrointestinal disorders (constipation, heartburn, hemorrhoids, etc.), the other was either a hospital control (acute orthopedic) or, in a few centers, a randomly chosen population control. Close to 500 patients and 1,000 controls were studied. The study attempted to evaluate perinatal factors, familial factors, diet, infections, vaccinations, allergic disorders, psychosomatic and social factors, etc. Preliminary results were presented at the XIIth International Congress of Gastroenterology in Lisbon, September, 1984. Lack of breast-feeding, the frequency of cereal consumption, infantile gastroenteritis and stressful life events in childhood did not discriminate between patients and controls. Final results of the study are still pending.

Comment

There is a great amount of indirect evidence pointing to the effect of environmental factors in IBD. These factors, however, have not yet been identified. The effect(s) of these putative factors on IBD is also uncertain. It may be causative, permissive or modulatory and it may particularly affect those in the population who are genetically predisposed. All this remains to be elucidated. It has to be emphasized that environmental and hereditary factors are *not* mutually exclusive. More likely both may be necessary for disease to develop.

At present there is an urgent need for direct studies to test the relevance to IBD of the various suggested factors. Doubtlessly, additional factors will be eventually suggested and will also have to be tested. It is to be hoped that eventually these studies will lead to the identification of the causative agent(s) of inflammatory bowel diseases.

References

1 Kyle, J.: An epidemiological study of Crohn's disease in Northeastern Scotland. Gastroenterology 61: 826–833 (1971).
2 Mendeloff, A. I.; Calkins, B. M.; Lilienfeld, A. M.; Garland, C. F.; Monk, M.: Inflammatory bowel disease in Baltimore, 1960–79. Hospital incidence rates, bimodality

and smoking factors; in McConnell, Rozen, Langman, Gilat, The genetics and epidemiology of inflammatory bowel disease, pp. 88–93 (Karger, Basel 1985).

3   Fahrlander, H.; Baerlocher C. H.: Clinical features and epidemiological data on Crohn's disease in the Basle area. Scand. J. Gastroent. 6: 657–662 (1971).

4   Mayberry, J.; Rhodes, J.; Hughes, L. E.: Incidence of Crohn's disease in Cardiff between 1934–1977. Gut 20: 602–608 (1973).

5   Binder, V.; Both, H.; Hansen, P. K.; Hendriksen, C.; Kreiner, S.; Torp-Pedersen, K.: Incidence and prevalence of ulcerative colitis and Crohn's disease in the county of Copenhagen, 1962 to 1978. Gastroenterology 83: 563–568 (1982).

6   Smith, I. S.; Young, S.; Gillespie, G.; O'Connor, J.; Bell, J. R.: Epidemiological aspects of Crohn's disease in Clydesdale 1961–70. Gut 16: 62–67 (1975).

7   Kewenter, J.; Hulten, L.; Kock, N. G.: The relationship and epidemiology of acute terminal ileitis and Crohn's disease. Gut 15: 801–804 (1974).

8   Brahme, F.; Lindstrom, C.; Wenckert A.: Crohn's disease in a defined population. An epidemiological study of incidence, prevalence, mortality, and secular trends in the city of Malmo, Sweden. Gastroenterology 69: 342 351 (1975).

9   Brandes, J. W.; Lorenz-Meyer, H.: Epidemiologische Aspekte zur Enterocolitis regionalis Crohn und Colitis ulcerosa in Marburg/Lahn (FRG) zwischen 1962 und 1975. Z. Gastroent. 21: 69 78 (1983).

10 Sedlack, R. E.; Whisnant, J.; Elveback, L. R.; Kurland, L. T.: Incidence of Crohn's disease in Olmsted County Minnesota, 1935–75. Am. J. Epidem. 112: 759–763 (1980).

11 Miller, D. S.; Keighley, A. C.; Langman, M. J. S.: Changing patterns in epidemiology of Crohn's disease Lancet ii. 691 693 (1974)

12 Hellers, G.: Crohn's disease in Stockholm County 1955–74. A study of epidemiology, results of surgical treatment and long-term prognosis. Acta chir. scand. 490: suppl., pp. 1–83 (1979).

13 Bergman, L.; Krause, U.: The incidence of Crohn's disease in central Sweden. Scand. J. Gastroent. 10: 725–729 (1975).

14 Rozen, P.; Zonis, J.; Yekutiel, P.; Gilat, T.: Crohn's disease in the Jewish population of Tel Aviv Yafo. Epidemiological and clinical aspects. Gastroenterology 76: 25–30 (1979).

15 Gilat, T.; Grossman, A.; Bujanover, Y.; Rozen, P.: Epidemiology of inflammatory bowel disease. State of the art and etiologic inferences; in Rachmilewitz, Developments in gastroenterology, vol. 3: Inflammatory bowel diseases, pp. 143–151 (Martinus Nijhoff, Hague 1982).

16 Kyle, J.: Epidemiology of Dalziel's disease. Programme and Abstracts, Int. Workshop Epidemiology and Genetics of Inflammatory Bowel Disease, Glaxo Laboratories, Symp., 1983, p. 52.

17 Lee, F. I.; Costello, F. T.: The changing incidence of Crohn's disease in Blackpool 1969–1983; in McConnell, Rozen, Langman, Gilat, The genetics and epidemiology of inflammatory bowel disease, pp. 102–113 (Karger, Basel 1985).

18 Ruiz Ochoa, V.; Potel, J.: Crohn's disease in Galicia, Spain 1976–1982; in McConnell, Rozen, Langman, Gilat, The genetics and epidemiology of inflammatory bowel disease, pp. 94–101 (Karger, Basel 1985).

19 Sinclair, T. S.; Brunt, P. W.; Mowat, N. A. G.: Nonspecific proctocolitis in northeastern Scotland. A community study. Gastroenterology 85: 1–11 (1983).

20 Wright, J. P.; Marks, I. N.; Jameson, C.; Garisch, J. A. M.; Burns, D. G., Kottler, R. E.: Inflammatory bowel disease in Cape Town, 1975–1980. I. Ulcerative colitis. S. Afr. med. J. 63: 223–226 (1983).

21 Eason, R. J.; Lee, S. P.; Tasman-Jones, C.: Inflammatory bowel disease in Auckland, New Zealand. Aust. N. Z. J. Med. 12: 125–131 (1982).

22   Devlin. H. B.; Datta. D.; Dellipiani, A. W.: The incidence and prevalence of in-
      flammatory bowel disease in North Tees health district. Wld J. Surg. *4:* 183–193
      (1980).
23   Hellers, G.; Berglund, M.; Brostrom, O.; Monsen, U.; Nordenstrom, J.; Nordenvall,
      B.; Sorstad, J.: The epidemiology of ulcerative colitis in Stockholm county 1955–79.
      Programme and Abstracts, Int. Workshop Epidemiology and Genetics of Inflamma-
      tory Bowel Disease, Glaxo Laboratories Symp., 1983, p. 52.
24   Gilat, T.; Ribak, J.; Benaroya, Y.; Zemishlany, Z.; Weissman, I.: Ulcerative colitis in
      the Jewish population of Tel-Aviv Jafo. Gastroenterology *66:* 335–342 (1974).
25   Wright, J. P.; Marks, I. N.; Jameson, C.; Garisch, J. A. M.; Burns, D. G., Kottler,
      R. E.: Inflammatory bowel disease in Cape Town, 1975–1980. II. Crohn's disease. S.
      Afr. med. J. *63:* 226–230 (1983).
26   Yamagata. S.: Crohn's disease in Japan: report of the Japanese Committee for Crohn's
      disease. Chairman Prof. S. Yamagata; in Lee, A global assessment of Crohn's disease,
      pp. 136–144 (Heyden, London 1981.)
27   Ng, M.: Inflammatory bowel diseases among Chinese in Hong Kong and China. Pro-
      gramme and Abstracts, Int. Workshop Epidemiology and Genetics of Inflammatory
      Bowel Disease, Glaxo Laboratories Symp., 1983, p. 41.
28   Couchman, K. G.; Wigley, R. D.: The distribution of the systematic connective tissue
      diseases, ulcerative colitis and Crohn's disease in New Zealand. An analysis of hospital
      admission statistics. N. Z. med. J. *74:* 231–233 (1973).
29   Lanfranchi, G. A.; Michelini, A.; Brignola, C.; Campieri, M.; Cortini, C.; Marzio, L.:
      Uno studio epidemiologico sulle malattie inflammatorie intestinali nella provincia di
      Bologna. G. clin. med. *57:* 235–245 (1976).
30   O'Donoghue, D. P.; Clark, M. L.: Inflammatory bowel disease in West Indians. Br.
      med. J. *iii:* 796 (1976).
31   Das, S. K.; Montgomery, R. D.: Chronic inflammatory bowel disease in Asian immi-
      grants. Pract. Med. *221:* 747–749 (1978).
32   Gilat, T.; Fireman, Z.; Grossman, A.; Rozen, P.: Inflammatory Bowel Disease in
      Jews; in McConnell, Rozen, Langman, Gilat, The genetics and epidemiology of in-
      flammatory bowel disease, pp. 135–140 (Karger, Basel 1985).
33   Humphreys, W. G.; Parks, T. G.: Crohn's disease in Northern Ireland. A retrospec-
      tive survey of 159 cases. Irish J. med. Sci. *144:* 437–446 (1975).
34   Mayberry, J. F.; Rhodes, J.; Newcombe, R. G.: Crohn's disease in Wales, 1967–1976.
      An epidemiological survey based on hospital admissions. Post-grad. med. J. *56:* 336–
      341 (1980).
35   Acheson, E. D.; Truelove, S. C.: Early weaning in the aetiology of ulcerative colitis.
      Br. med. J. *ii:* 929–933 (1961).
36   Bergstrand, O.; Hellers, G.: Breast feeding during infancy in patients who later de-
      velop Crohn's disease. Scand. J. Gastroent. *18:* 903–906 (1983).
37   Whorwell, P. J.; Holdstock, G.; Whorwell, G. M.; Wright, R.: Bottle feeding, early
      gastroenteritis and inflammatory bowel disease. Br. med. J. *i:* 382 (1979).
38   Martini, G. A.; Brandes, J. W.: Increased consumption of refined carbohydrates in
      patients with Crohn's disease. Klin. Wschr. *54:* 367–371 (1976).
39   Silkoff, A.; Hallak, A.; Yegena, L.; Rozen, P.; Mayberry, J. F.; Rhodes, J.; New-
      combe, R. G.: Consumption of refined carbohydrate by patients with Crohn's disease
      in Tel Aviv-Jafo. Post-grad. med. J. *56:* 28–32 (1980).
40   Mayberry, J. F.; Rhodes, J.; Newcombe, R. G.: Increased sugar consumption in
      Crohn's disease. Digestion *20:* 323–326 (1980).
41   Thornton, J. R.; Emmett, P. M.; Heaton, K. W.: Diet and Crohn's disease; character-
      istics of the pre-illness diet. Br. med. J. *ii:* 762–764 (1979).

42   Kasper, H.; Sommer, H.: Dietary fibre and nutrient intake in Crohn's disease. Am. J. clin. Nutr. *32:* 1898–1901 (1979).

43   Jarnerot, G.; Jarnmar, K. I.; Nilsson, K.: Consumption of refined sugar by patients with Crohn's disease, ulcerative colitis or irritable bowel syndrome. Scand. J. Gastroent. *18:* 999–1002 (1983).

44   Penny, W. J.; Mayberry, J. F.; Aggett, P. J.; Gilbert, J. O.; Newcombe, R. G.; Rhodes, J. M.: Relationship between trace elements, sugar consumption, and taste in Crohn's disease. Gut *24:* 288–292 (1983).

45   Kasper, H.; Sommer, H.: Taste thresholds in patients with Crohn's disease. J. hum. Nutr. *34:* 455–456 (1980).

46   Tiomny, E.; Horwitz, C.; Graff, E.; Rozen, P.; Gilat, T.: Serum zinc and taste acuity in Tel Aviv patients with inflammatory bowel disease. Am. J. Gastroent. *77:* 101–104 (1982).

47   James, A. H.: Breakfast and Crohn's disease. Br. med. J. *i:* 943–945 (1977).

48   Rawcliffe, P. M.; Truelove, S. C.: Breakfast and Crohn's disease. Br. med. J. *iii:* 539–540 (1978).

49   Archer, L. N. J.; Harvey, R. F.; Breakfast and Crohn's disease. Br. med. J. *iii:* 540 (1978).

50   Guthy, E.: Morbus Crohn and Nahrungsfette. Dt. med. Wschr. *107:* 71–73 (1982).

51   Sachar, D. B.: Animal transmission models. Mount Sinai J. Med. *50:* 166–170 (1983).

52   Dourmashkin, R. R.: Microbiologic approaches. Mount Sinai J. Med. *50:* 171–177 (1983).

53   Gutensohn, N.; Cole, P.. Childhood social environment and Hodgkin's disease. New Engl. J. Med. *304:* 135–140 (1981).

54   Miller, D. S.; Keighley, A.; Smith, P. G; Hughes, A. O.; Langman, M. J. S.: Crohn's disease in Nottingham: A search for time-space clustering. Gut *16:* 454–457 (1975).

55   Rhodes, J. M.; Cockel, R.; Allan, R. N.; Hawker, P. C.; Dawson, J.; Elias, E.: Colonic Crohn's disease and use of oral contraception. Br. med. J. *288:* 595–596 (1984).

56   Harries, A. D.; Baird, A.; Rhodes. J.: Non-smoking. A feature of ulcerative colitis. Br. med. J. *284:* 706 (1982).

57   Jick, J.; Walker, A. M.: Cigarette smoking and ulcerative colitis. New Engl. J. Med. *308:* 261–263 (1983).

58   Logan, R. F. A.; Edmond, M.; Somerville, K. W.; Langman, M. J. S.: Smoking and ulcerative colitis. Br. med. J. *288:* 751–753 (1984).

59   Somerville, K. W.; Logan, R. F. A.; Edmond, E. M.; Langman, M. J. S.: Smoking and Crohn's disease. Br. med. J. *289:* 954–956 (1984).

60   Cantor, D. S.: Crohn's disease and psychiatric illness. Gastroenterology *87:* 478–479 (1984).

T. Gilat, MD, Department of Gastroenterology, Ichilov Hospital,
Tel Aviv 64239 (Israel)

Subject Index